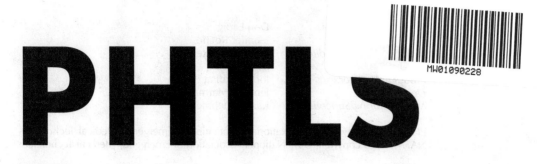

PHTLS

BASIC AND
ADVANCED
PREHOSPITAL TRAUMA LIFE SUPPORT

Instructor's Manual
Fourth Edition

Developed by the National Association of
Emergency Medical Technicians
in cooperation with
The Committee on Trauma
of the American College of Surgeons

International PHTLS Office
408 Monroe Street
Clinton, Mississippi 39056
1-800-94-PHTLS

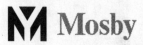

St. Louis Baltimore Boston Carlsbad Chicago Naples New York Philadelphia Portland
London Madrid Mexico City Singapore Sydney Tokyo Toronto Wiesbaden

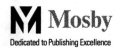
Mosby
Dedicated to Publishing Excellence

Publisher:	Don Ladig
Executive Editor:	Jennifer Roche
Sr. Developmental Editor:	Kellie F. White
Project Manager:	Mark Spann
Production Editor:	Jodi Everding
Designer:	Jennifer Marmarinos
Manufacturing Supervisor:	Karen Boehme

PHTLS logo copyright © by National Association of Emergency Medical Technicians
NAEMT logo copyright © by National Association of Emergency Medical Technicians

Fourth Edition

Copyright © 1999 by Mosby, Inc.

Previous editions copyrighted 1986, 1990 by Educational Direction, Inc., Akron, Ohio and 1994 by Mosby–Year Book, Inc.

Printed in the United States of America

Composition by Graphic World, Inc.
Printing/Binding by Plus Communications, Inc.

Mosby, Inc.
11830 Westline Industrial Drive
St. Louis, Missouri 63146

International Standard Book Number 0-3230-0300-1

Contributors

EDITOR-IN-CHIEF

Norman E. McSwain, Jr., MD, FACS, NREMT-P
Professor of Surgery
Tulane University School of Medicine
New Orleans, Louisiana

CONTRIBUTORS

Ann Bellows, RN, NREMT-P, EdD
Training Specialist
Doña Ana Branch Community College
New Mexico State University
Las Cruces, New Mexico

Will Chapleau, EMT-P, RN, TNS, CEN
Chairman, PHTLS
Emergency Medical Services Coordinator
Emergency Medical Education
St. James Hospital
Chicago, Illinois

Gregory Chapman, RRT, REMT-P
Certified Instructor Coordinator
Institute of Prehospital Emergency Medicine
Hudson Valley Community College
Troy, New York

Scott Frame, MD, FACS, FCCM
Associate Professor of Surgery
Director, Division of Trauma/Critical Care
University of Cincinnati Medical Center
Cincinnati, Ohio

Steve Mercer, EMT-P
Education Coordinator
Iowa Department of Public Health
Bureau of Emergency Medical Services
Des Moines, Iowa

Preface

With this Instructor Manual we have attempted to produce a tool for our instructors that will assist them in conducting any of our PHTLS programs. We have also tried to put it together in such a manner that would create a reference tool for our faculty to be used as a quick reference for any questions an Instructor may have about PHTLS policies and course materials.

The PHTLS Executive Council created the fourth edition materials using current educational practice and also in response to comments and specific requests from our faculty all over the world. As the PHTLS program is always evolving, responding to the changes in medicine and in particular, prehospital care, we are also interested in feedback about our materials.

Please feel free to contact us through the National office if you have comments you'd like to share with us about the Instructor Manual or any of the Program Support materials.

PHTLS Education Committee
PHTLS Executive Council
PHTLS International headquarters
408 Monroe Street
Clinton, Mississippi 39056
1-800-94-PHTLS
fax: 601-924-7325
e-mail: NAEMTHQ@AOL.COM

DISCLAIMER STATEMENT

A NOTE TO THE READER: The authors and publisher have made every attempt to ensure that the guidelines presented in this text are accurate and represent accepted practices in the United States. They are not provided as a standard of care. EMS providers perform procedures under the authority of a licensed physician. It is the reader's responsibility to follow patient care protocols established by a medical direction physician and to remain current in the delivery of emergency care. The procedures presented in this text fall within the philosophies of the American College of Surgeons, Committee on Trauma (ACS-COT) as set forth in the Advanced Trauma Life Support (ATLS) course.

Introduction

Prehospital Trauma Life Support (PHTLS) courses are nationally recognized continuing education programs for prehospital emergency health care professionals that bring the care of the trauma patient into a single focus. Previous training has been notable for fragmenting our approach to, and understanding of, the trauma patient as a single entity.

PHTLS courses provide a prehospital trauma care philosophy, stressing the need to treat the multisystem trauma patient as a unique entity with specific needs. This may require an approach to the trauma patient that varies from traditional treatment modalities.

PHTLS courses are based on the Advanced Trauma Life Support (ATLS), a course for physicians developed by the American College of Surgeons Committee on Trauma. More importantly, PHTLS courses follow the protocols for prehospital care of trauma patients as developed by the committee on trauma.

The Committee on Trauma of the American College of Surgeons provides the medical direction and content oversight for the PHTLS program. They are represented by the medical directors on the Executive Council of the PHTLS Division of the National Association of EMTs.

The National Association of Emergency Medical Technicians (NAEMT) was founded in 1975, with support from the National Registry of EMTs and other leaders in emergency medicine. The NAEMT mission is to ensure a professional representative organization to represent the views and opinions of prehospital personnel and thus to influence the future advancement of EMTs as health care professionals. Additionally, the NAEMT serves its membership through educational programs (such as PHTLS), liaison activities, working toward development of national standards and reciprocity, and other activities to benefit EMTs.

Since it was founded, the NAEMT has developed numerous liaison relationships with federal and state level agencies and professional organizations representing emergency medicine and public safety interests. The American College of Surgeons, American College of Emergency Physicians, National Registry of EMTs, Commission on Accreditation of Ambulance Services, Emergency Nurses Association, and the National EMS Alliance are but a few of the organizations with whom the NAEMT has liaison relationships.

The PHTLS Division of NAEMT serves as a valuable resource to the President and Board of Governors of NAEMT. The Division work process begins with the establishment of objectives by the PHTLS Division Executive Council. The PHTLS Executive Council submits regular reports to the NAEMT President for review by the NAEMT Board of Directors.

The PHTLS Executive Council is responsible for the design, conduct, and dissemination of the course. The International Advisory Council, a multidisciplinary group of health care professionals with an interest in EMS, review and comment on PHTLS materials and activities.

Through the Chairperson, the PHTLS Executive Council appoints and oversees the performance of International, National, and affiliate faculty, as well as the Regional and State Coordinators. The Division Chairperson reports to the President of NAEMT. The Committee on Trauma of the American College of Surgeons is permanently represented on the Executive Council by the PHTLS Medical Directors.

This Instructor Manual has been prepared to inform potential course sponsors and Instructor/Coordinators of the program's purpose, organizational structure, course requirements, and lecture outlines. Each PHTLS course must be approved and conducted as prescribed in the Instructor Manual with the involvement of the appropriate NAEMT/PHTLS personnel and the State/Provincial Committee on Trauma Chair (or designee).

GOALS AND OBJECTIVES

The primary goals of Prehospital Trauma Life Support are as follows:

- To provide a description of the physiology and kinematics of injury.

- To provide an understanding of the need for a rapid assessment of the trauma patient.

- To advance the participant's level of knowledge in regard to examination and diagnostic skills.

- To enhance the participant's performance in the assessment and treatment of the trauma patient.

- To advance the participant's level of competence in regard to specific prehospital trauma intervention skills.

- To provide an overview and establish a management method for the prehospital care of the multisystem trauma patient.

The PHTLS course is designed to provide the practicing prehospital care provider with a specific body of knowledge related to the prehospital assessment and care of the trauma patient. It is stressed that this is a continuing education program and contains information that may be a review for some or all participants. The uniqueness of this program rests not with an entirely new body of knowledge but instead with advances in prehospital trauma intervention techniques. We are using new combinations and applications of existing skills and knowledge to better our patients' chances at surviving traumatic events.

PHTLS TRAINING PROGRAMS

The PHTLS Executive Council would like to stress that safety is a very important issue when conducting these courses. Be sure that you create a safe atmosphere for your course participants and faculty to work in.

PROVIDER COURSE

PHTLS has always been a scenario-based program. With this edition of the instructor materials, we have further enhanced the scenario's role in the lecture format. This enhancement is the result of feedback and comments from our instructors.

The PHTLS Provider course is designed to be an intensive 16-hour experience. It is available to all levels of prehospital care providers.

The lecture and skill station content is designed for a course that is taught in a time frame of approximately 17 hours. The arrangement of lectures and interactive skill stations is deliberate. No shortening of this time is allowable. Time frame alterations, however, may be appropriate in some circumstances based on the skill level of the participants.

The intracurricular program may be integrated into the Emergency Medical Technician-Basic, EMT-Intermediate, EMT-Paramedic, or equivalent program after approval by the Regional or State Coordinator. Courses within EMT-Basic programs must be presented at the conclusion of the course.

INSTRUCTOR COURSE

The PHTLS Instructor/Coordinator Workshop is designed to be an intensive 8-hour course for those individuals who have already successfully completed a PHTLS provider course. A 3-day version is available, combining provider and instructor components.

This course is designed to train instructor candidates for conducting provider and refresher courses on the latest philosophies and techniques. Individuals selected to attend this workshop will typically be experienced instructors, coordinators, or administrators with proven clinical skills at a minimum of the EMT-Basic level.

REFRESHER COURSE

The PHTLS Refresher course is designed to be an 8-hour workshop. It is offered at the basic and advanced levels and incorporates interactive teaching sessions and evaluation stations. Candidates who wish to participate in a refresher course must have successfully completed a PHTLS or BTLS provider course within the last 3 years prior to the course.

Recognition of successful completion for PHTLS Provider and Refresher courses is for 3 years.

INSTRUCTOR UPDATE

The PHTLS textbook, Instructor Manual, and slide set are in a continuous review and update process that is linked to the ATLS materials. There will be new, updated course materials published every 4 years, approximately 1 year after the new ATLS materials are released. Instructors that wish to run courses using the new materials will be required to first attend a PHTLS Instructor update workshop. These will be conducted by PHTLS National faculty and disseminated through the affiliates under the guidance of the

PHTLS Executive Council. There will be a limited phase-in period during which the previous edition will still be available for instructors who have not attended an update. Upon release of the new materials, the dates for update courses will be distributed along with notification on how long the previous edition will be available.

COURSE MATERIALS

PHTLS Provider Textbook

The required text for this program is the *Prehospital Trauma Life Support—Fourth Edition*. This textbook is written by the National Association of Emergency Medical Technicians and published by Mosby, Inc., 1998. The book is an important and required part of the program, but it is only a single component of the PHTLS program. Interactive exercises, written and practical evaluations, and lectures reinforce the content of the textbook.

PHTLS Instructor Manual

This PHTLS Instructor Manual contains the NAEMT/PHTLS Division requirements for successful course completion, description of the PHTLS organization, outline of the faculty responsibilities, and program guidelines. All PHTLS faculty must adhere to these requirements. It also contains lecture content material and descriptions of the skill stations and the equipment needed to run them.

PHTLS Slides

The PHTLS slides, covering all of the PHTLS courses, are copyrighted material. No reproduction of these slides is permitted in any form. Slides may be purchased by approved PHTLS Course Coordinators. Authorization for purchase of slides can be obtained from the National office upon recommendation of State or National faculty. Once purchased, the purchaser agrees to use the slides only in approved PHTLS courses and to not duplicate them in any manner.

If the slides are not purchased, one set will be loaned to approved course sites for approved courses. The application for the course must be received at least 30 days in advance of the course, and the slides must be returned to the International PHTLS office within 2 weeks after the end of the course.

If a course site has not received the slides within 21 days of the course, the Course Coordinator should contact the International PHTLS office.

Contents

Contents

SECTION I

Provider Program

LESSON 1

Introduction

OBJECTIVES

At the completion of this course, participants will be able to:
- Demonstrate an understanding of the kinematics of trauma.
- Establish and execute priorities of care in multisystem trauma situations.
- Demonstrate the basic skills that are key to prehospital management of trauma patients.

Setting

The course should be conducted in facilities that are well lit and comfortable with opportunity for realistic scenarios and with adequate space to perform.

Time

The provider course must be at least 16 hours in length. The optimum experience is the 2-day, 8 hours per day method. The course can also be split up over 3 or 4 days. Course quality suffers when it is extended much beyond these parameters.

Materials

Each course participant must have a textbook made available to them prior to the course. We recommend that the participants receive the book at least 2 weeks before the course.

Instructors

Ideally your entire faculty should be trained PHTLS Instructors. The minimum number for the course to be approved is four. The number of instructors will have to be increased to accommodate larger classes.

PHTLS PROVIDER COURSE SCHEDULE

The schedule provided here is for the 2-day course.

Day One

7:30 am	Registration
8:00 am	Introductions
8:10 am	Baseline Determinations
9:40 am	Course Purpose
9:55 am	Kinematics
10:45 am	Break
11:00 am	Patient Assessment
11:50 am	Airway Management
12:20 pm	Lunch
1:05 pm	Shock and Fluid Replacement
1:50 pm	Spinal Trauma
2:20 pm	Assessment Demonstration Video
2:35 pm	Practical Skill Stations
5:35 pm	Reassemble/Recess

Day Two

8:00 am	Considerations in the Pediatric and Elderly Patient
8:30 am	Thoracic Trauma
9:00 am	Abdominal Trauma and Trauma in Pregnancy
9:20 am	Break
9:35 am	Head Trauma
10:10 am	Practical Skills Teaching Stations
11:10 am	Musculoskeletal Trauma
11:25 am	Thermal Trauma
11:55 am	Lunch
12:40 pm	Essentials in Prehospital Care
12:55 pm	Final Assessment
3:55 pm	Reassemble/Summation, Adjourn

Slide No.	Lecture Content	Notes

1-1 *Title Slide*

1-2 *Development of PHTLS Program: NAEMT, COT/ASC, Mosby*

1-3 *Provider Course Objectives*

FOCUS: **Review objectives**

- Rapid and accurate assessment to determine the presence or potential for life threats
- Identification of shock and hypoxemia
- Initiation of intervention techniques
- Rapid and safe transport

At the end of this course participants should be able to identify shock and hypoxemia in the early as well as the late stages, know when and where intervention techniques must occur to provide the patient the best care, and initiate appropriate transport based on patient condition with intervention en route as indicated.

1-4 *Have You Seen This Scenario Before?*

FOCUS: **Baselines**

This is the baseline scenario.

1-5 *Purpose of PHTLS Baselines*

FOCUS: **Discuss and briefly review the performances at baselines**

- Identify areas for improvement.
- Rapidly determine potential life-threatening injuries and priorities.
- Develop a team approach.

Give a brief summary of general problem areas. Encourage group to provide examples, i.e., mechanism; hypoxemia and hypovolemia life threats; key to oxygenate, rapidly extricate, transport, give IVs en route. Remind students that it requires the whole team working as a unit to accomplish the goals.

1-6 *PHTLS History*

1-7 FOCUS: **Brief overview of the history of PHTLS**

- Developed in response to a need for improved prehospital trauma care
- Developed by the National Association of EMTs (NAEMT) in cooperation with the American College of Surgeons (ACS)
- PHTLS has become a recognized standard in the prehospital management of trauma patients.

Slide No.	Lecture Content	Notes

- PHTLS has been adopted by international medical communities and is currently being offered in many foreign countries.

In the past, EMS providers stayed in the field to immobilize all trauma patients, thus decreasing the chance for patients to receive definitive care within the "golden hour." PHTLS encouraged rapid identification, assessment, and management of critical trauma patients with an emphasis on decreasing scene times.

1-8   *Epidemiology of Trauma*

1-9   FOCUS: **Identify the seriousness of trauma**

- Trauma is the leading cause of death in patients aged from 1 to 44 years old.
- Trauma is the third leading cause of death in all age groups.
- More than 60 million injuries occur annually in the United States alone.
- Trauma is a major problem worldwide.
- Besides its direct costs, trauma also causes lost tax income, lost productivity, and lost years of life.

Supplement with any local or regional statistics.

1-10   *Death, Disability, and Intervention*

FOCUS: **How EMS impacts death from trauma**

How can EMS make a difference?

- Death in the first hour
- Death in the first 4 hours
- Death in 6 weeks

EMS can provide injury prevention education, as the only chance some patients have is for the incident to not have occurred. EMS can make a difference through timely appropriate care to reduce mortality and morbidity. EMS can communicate index of suspicion to increase the chance for appropriate response of the trauma system.

1-11   *Trauma Is Staged Death*

FOCUS: **Remind students that shock progresses to death in an orderly fashion**

R. Adams Cowley identified the "golden hour." He found that patients suffering from major trauma had a higher survival rate if surgical intervention (definitive care) occurred within 1 hour of insult.

From this golden hour, EMS has allocated a platinum 10 minutes, or less, as the ideal scene time to optimize the chance of patients receiving definitive care in the first hour.

Recognition of the early stages of shock allows the EMS provider to determine which patients are unstable or **potentially unstable**, needing rapid transport, and which patients can be managed on scene for a longer period of time.

Slide No.	Lecture Content	Notes

1-12   *Trauma Team—Golden Hour*

FOCUS: **Review the members of the team necessary to make the golden hour work**

The trauma team participants during the golden hour include:
- Prehospital responders
- Transport services
- Emergency department
- Operating suite

The team must be prepared, have a system in place, and communicate with each other in order to optimize the golden hour for critical trauma patients.

1-13   *Trauma Centers*

FOCUS: **Why trauma centers work**
- In-house surgical team
- Operating room available
- Expertise in dealing with traumatized patients
- Access to critical care and rehabilitation

Trauma centers provide immediate access to definitive care for critical trauma patients. Discuss alternatives if trauma centers are not available in the area of the course.

1-14   *The Platinum 10 Minutes*

FOCUS: **Activities that must occur within the platinum 10 minutes**
- Identification of critical patients
- Assessment and treatment of life-threatening injuries
- Rapid extrication where indicated
- Timely transport to an appropriate facility
- Early alerting of the receiving facility

1-15   *Most Important*

FOCUS: **The patient as the most important person**
- Who is the most important person in trauma?

The patient is the most important person in trauma.

1-16   *Trauma Care*

FOCUS: **Critical trauma patients need surgery and interventions that cannot occur in the field**
- What is the definitive care for trauma?
- What is our goal in the severely injured trauma patient?

Definitive care is surgical intervention and resuscitation to control hemorrhage or hypoxemia. Our goal is to get the patient to definitive care as efficiently as possible while completing the appropriate prehospital assessment and management of life threats.

Slide No.	Lecture Content	Notes

1-17

Components of PHTLS

FOCUS: **Brief overview of the components of the course**

- Lectures
- Hands-on skill stations
- Final scenarios
- Final written evaluation

PHTLS presents lectures on trauma topics ranging from kinematics to burns. Hands-on skill stations cover airway management, patient assessment, spinal immobilization, helmet removal, and rapid extrication. Final scenarios require hands-on assessment and care of a simulated patient. The interaction and reinforcement of all of these components help direct students to work as a unified group to improve prehospital care of the trauma patient.

1-18

Introduction Summary

FOCUS: **Key to lecture**

Trauma care is the area in which YOU can make the largest impact on the patient's *final outcome.*

Kinematics

CHAPTER OBJECTIVES

At the completion of this course the student will be able to:

- Define energy and force as they relate to trauma.

- Define laws of motion energy and undersand the geometric role increased speed plays in causing injuries.

- Describe each type of auto collision and its effect on unrestrained victims (e.g., "down-and-under," "up-and-over," compression, deceleration).

- Describe the pathophysiology of the head, spine, thorax, and abdomen that result from the above named forces.

- List specific injuries and their causes as related to interior and exterior vehicle damage.

- Describe the function of supplemental restraint systems (air bags).

- Describe the kinematics of penetrating injuries.

- List the motion and energy considerations of mechanisms other than motor vehicle collisions (e.g., blasts, falls).

- Define the role of kinematics as an additional tool for patient assessment.

Slide No.	Lecture Content	Notes

2-1 A   *Title Slides*

2-1 B

2-2   *Lesson 2 Objectives*

FOCUS: **Review objectives**

- Discuss the laws of energy and motion.
- Discuss trauma associated with blunt impact and penetrating trauma.
- Overview of the effects of energy distribution in MVCs.
- Review the kinematics of blast and violent injuries.
- Use kinematics to predict injury patterns.

2-3   *Kinetic Energy*

FOCUS: **Describe the formula for kinetic energy**

$$KE = \frac{mass\ (weight) \times velocity\ (speed)^2}{2}$$

Or

$$KE = \frac{mv^2}{2}$$

Kinetic energy is the energy of motion

2-4   *Example of Kinetic Energy*

FOCUS: **Apply the kinetic energy formula to a patient**

- The KE of a 150-lb person traveling at 30 mph would be:

$$\frac{150 \times 30 \times 30}{2} = 67,500\ KE\ units$$

2-5   *Velocity vs. Mass*

FOCUS: **Apply the kinetic energy formula to patients**

- 150-lb person traveling at 30 mph = 67,500 KE uits
- 180-lb person traveling at 30 mph = 81,000 KE units
- 150-lb person traveling at 40 mph = 120,000 KE units

What is more important: velocity or mass?

2-6   *Velocity*

FOCUS: **Velocity has a greater influence than mass on the production of kinetic energy**

2-7   *Newton's First Law of Motion*

FOCUS: **Identifying Newton's First Law of Motion**

- A body at rest will stay at rest.
- A body in motion will remain in motion.
- Unless what?

A body in motion will remain in motion unless it is acted on by an outside force.

Slide No.	Lecture Content	Notes

2-8   *Newton's First Law and Blunt Trauma*

FOCUS: **Apply Newton's First Law of Motion to a trauma patient**

- Car strikes pole
- Driver continues moving forward
- Anterior surface of body strikes steering wheel
- Posterior body continues moving forward
- Organs compressed within body

2-9   *Law of Conservation of Energy*

FOCUS: **Understand the Law of Conservation of Energy**

- Energy cannot be created.
- Energy cannot be destroyed.
- Energy *can* change forms and can be transferred.
- Can you give an example?

Example: As a driver applies the brakes in a car, the brakes cause friction. This causes a change in the form of energy to heat.

2-10   *Law of Conservation of Energy*

FOCUS: **Applying the Law of Conservation of Energy to a trauma patient**

- How does the Law of Conservation of Energy pertain to trauma?
- Can you give some examples?

2-11   *Deceleration and Acceleration*

2-12   FOCUS: **Compression/shear of internal organs**

- Compression injury
- Shear injury

2-13   *Organ Injury*

FOCUS: **Identifying coup and contra-coup injuries**

In a 50-mph MVC, what types of injuries would occur if the patient were to strike the windshield?

2-14   *Head and Neck Injury*

FOCUS: **Identifying damage associated with head and neck injuries**

- Fractures
- Ligamentous injuries
- Soft tissue injury
- Brain injury
- Cord damage

Slide No.	Lecture Content	Notes

2-15 *Torso Injury*
FOCUS: **Identifying damage associated with torso injuries**
- Rib fractures
- Heart and lung damage
- Abdominal organ damage
- Major vessel damage

2-16 *Extremity Injury*
FOCUS: **Identifying damage associated with extremity injuries**
- Fractures
- Ligamentous injury
- Soft tissue injury

2-17 *Types of Motor Vehicle Collisions*
FOCUS: **Identifying the five types of vehicle collisions**
- Frontal impact
- Lateral impact
- Rotational impact
- Rear impact
- Rollover

2-18 *Picture of Frontal Impact*
FOCUS: **Identifying injuries associated with frontal impacts**
What type of injury patterns might you see in a frontal impact?

2-19 *Frontal Impact—Occupant Pathways*
FOCUS: **Identifying up-and-over pathway injuries**
- What injuries would you expect with an up-and-over pathway?

2-20 *Injuries with Up-and-Over Pathway*
2-21 FOCUS: **Types of injuries associated with up-and-over pathway**
- Head injuries
- Spine injuries
- Chest injuries
  - Fractures
  - Pneumothorax
  - Hemothorax
  - Contusions
  - Great vessel injury
- Abdominal injuries
  - Solid organs
  - Hollow organs
  - Diaphragm
- Fractured pelvis

Slide No.	Lecture Content	Notes

2-22   *Frontal Impact—Occupant Pathways*

FOCUS: **Identifying injuries associated with down-and-under pathway**

What injuries would you expect?

2-23   *Injuries with Down-and-Under Pathway*

FOCUS: **Injuries associated with down-and-under pathway**

- Posterior knee/hip dislocations
- Femur fractures
- Lower extremity fractures
- Pelvic/acetabular fractures

2-24   *Rear Impact*

FOCUS: **Identifying injuries associated with rear impact collisions**

What types of injuries would you expect with this type of impact?

2-25   *Lateral Impact*

FOCUS: **Identifying injuries associated with lateral impact collisions**

What types of injuries would you expect with a lateral impact collision?

2-26   *Body Motion during Lateral Impacts*

FOCUS: **Understanding the body's movement during a lateral impact**

- Neck
- Chest
- Pelvis

2-27   *Rotational Impact*

FOCUS: **Discuss injuries associated with rotational impact**

What type of injuries would you expect with a rotational impact?

2-28   *Rollover*

FOCUS: **Discuss injuries associated with vehicle rollovers**

What injury patterns might you see following this collision?

Slide No.	Lecture Content	Notes

2-29

Lap Restraint Device

FOCUS: **Identify injuries associated with the use of properly and improperly positioned lap restraints when the driver or passenger is involved in a collision**

- Properly positioned lap restraint
- Improperly positioned lap restraint

What types of injuries should you anticipate?

- Lap restraints work best when used in conjunction with shoulder restraints.
- The upper body may rotate into the steering wheel or other vehicle structures when a lap restraint is used alone.
- Improperly positioned lap restraints (too high/too low) may cause internal organ damage.

2-30

Lap and Shoulder Restraint System

FOCUS: **Identify injury patterns associated with improperly used restraint devices**

- Shoulder harness only; lap belt not used
  - (Victim moves down and under.)
- Lap restraint only; shoulder harness not used
  - (Victim moves up and over.)
- What types of injuries should you anticipate?

Shoulder restraints must be used with lap restraints.

2-31

Air Bag Deployment

FOCUS: **Identifying injuries associated with air bag deployment**

- What types of injuries would you expect to see?
- What injuries would occur in a second collision?

Air bag deployment alone will not prevent serious injuries. Air bags work best with lap and shoulder restraints. If a second collision occurs after deployment of the air bag, the risk of serious injuries increases. Remember to check under the deployed air bag for vehicle structure damage.

2-32

Air Bag Deployment

FOCUS: **Discuss injuries associated with air bag deployment**

- What concerns would you have about a:
  - Small patient?
  - Child in a car seat?

Air bag deployment may cause severe or fatal injuries in small patients and children in car seats.

Slide No.	Lecture Content	Notes

2-33   *Motorcycle Collisions*

FOCUS: **Discuss local helmet laws and how helmets decrease mortality and morbidity**

Mandatory helmet laws have been associated with a decrease in head injuries and deaths by up to 300%.

2-34   *Types of Impacts*

2-35   FOCUS: **Identify injuries associated with different types of motorcycle collisions**

- Frontal/ejection
- Lateral

How many impacts will occur for each type of collision? What types of injuries would you expect to see?

2-36   *Pedestrian vs. Motor Vehicle*

FOCUS: **Identify injuries associated with adults and children if struck by a motor vehicle**

How would the injury patterns differ between the adult and the child?

- Adults will generally turn away from an oncoming vehicle while a child will turn and face the vehicle.
- An adult's injuries will tend to be limited to the lower extremities and head injuries from striking the pavement.
- A child's injuries can be more severe due to the height of the vehicle in relationship to the height of the child (i.e., chest and abdominal injuries).

2-37   *Falls*

FOCUS: **The nature and severity of injuries from falls are related to the height of the fall and the surface on which the individual lands**

- Impact surface
  - Harder surface = greater injury
- Height
  - Greater height = greater injury
- Falls from a distance of more than three times the patient's height produce critical injuries

2-38   *Falls*

FOCUS: **Discuss deceleration injuries to internal organs from falls**

Deceleration injuries:

- Liver
- Aorta
- Spleen
- Kidney

Slide No.	Lecture Content	Notes

2-39 *Landing Feet First (Don Juan Syndrome)*

FOCUS: **Discuss injuries associated with patients landing feet first from a fall**

Injuries seen in patients landing feet first:

- Bilateral heel fractures
- Ankle fractures
- Distal tibia/fibula fractures
- Knee dislocations
- Femur fractures
- Hip injuries
- Spine compression fractures

2-40 *Landing Arms/Hands First*

FOCUS: **Discuss injuries associated with patients landing arms/hands first from a fall**

Physical findings:

- Colles fractures of the wrists
- Shoulder dislocations
- Fractures of the clavicles

2-41 *Landing Head First*

FOCUS: **Discuss injuries associated with patients landing head first from a fall**

Physical findings:

- Cervical spine injuries
- Facial injuries
- CNS damage

2-42 *Sports and Recreational Activity Mechanisms*

FOCUS: **Discuss mechanism of injuries associated with sporting and recreational activities**

- Acceleration
- Deceleration
- Hyperextension
- Hyperflexion
- Twisting
- Falling

What types of sporting or recreational injuries are common to your area?

2-43 *Predicting Sports-related Injuries*

FOCUS: **Discuss factors that should be evaluated when dealing with a sports-related injury**

- Kinematics and forces involved
- Equipment contributing to injury
- Involvement of protective equipment
- Nature of the sport

Slide No.	Lecture Content	Notes

2-44   *Blast Injuries*

FOCUS: **Discuss common locations for potential explosions**

- Warfare
- Civilian areas
  - Mines
  - Shipyards
  - Chemical plants
  - Tank trucks
  - Refineries
  - Fireworks firms
  - Silos
  - LP gas tanks

Do you have any of these in your area?

    The incidence of blast injuries increases during warfare, but these injuries are also becoming more common in the civilian world.

2-45   *Blast-related Injuries*

FOCUS: **Discuss the three phases of a blast and its related injuries**

Three mechanisms of injury:

- Primary
- Secondary
- Tertiary

2-46   *Primary Phase Injuries*

FOCUS: **Discuss the cause of injury and the types of injuries sustained from the primary phase of a blast**

- Cause: Pressure wave from blast
- Affected area: Gas-containing organs
- Injuries:
  - Pulmonary bleeding
  - Pneumothorax
  - Air emboli
  - Perforation of the GI tract
  - Burns

Death may occur in absence of outward signs.

2-47   *Secondary Phase Injuries*

FOCUS: **Discuss the cause of injury and the types of injuries sustained from the secondary phase of a blast**

- Cause: Flying debris
- Affected area:
  - Body surface
  - Skeletal system
- Injuries:
  - Lacerations
  - Fractures
  - Burns

Slide No.	Lecture Content	Notes

2-48

Tertiary Phase Injuries

FOCUS: **Discuss the cause of injury and the types of injuries sustained from the tertiary phase of a blast**

- Cause: Victim thrown against an object
- Affected area: Area of impact or referred energy
- Injuries: Similar to those sustained in a vehicle ejection

2-49

Penetrating Trauma

FOCUS: **Introduction to penetrating injuries section and areas that will be discussed**

- Physics
- Weapon velocity
- Bullet design

2-50

Penetrating Trauma

FOCUS: **Discuss transfer of energy**

Newton's First Law and ballistics:

- Bullet in brass cartridge is at rest.
- Bullet propelled by rapid combustion of powder.
- Bullet leaves barrel of gun.
- Bullet strikes a body.
- Bullet transfers energy to victim.

The chemical energy changes to heat then to motion then to injury.

2-51

Low-energy Injuries

FOCUS: **Discuss cause and effects from low-energy injuries**

- Low velocity
- Usually hand-driven weapons
- Less secondary trauma
- Multiple wounds from a single weapon

A knife, ice pick, and scissors are common weapons causing low-energy injuries. Injuries are usually limited to the depth and area of penetration.

2-52

Low-energy Penetrating Wounds

FOCUS: **Discuss the area of coning (tissue damage) produced with low-energy penetrating injuries**

- Would a longer knife leave a larger cone of damage?

Longer weapons increase the potential for greater depth and a greater area of damage.

Slide No.	Lecture Content	Notes

2-53

Assessment of Low-energy Injuries

FOCUS: **Discuss areas of special attention during assessment of low-energy penetrating injuries**

- Type of weapon involved
- Path of weapon
- Depth of penetration
- Number of wounds
- Underlying anatomy

2-54

Medium-energy Penetrating Injuries

FOCUS: **Discuss injury patterns associated with medium-energy weapons**

- Injuries similar to low-energy penetrating injuries
- More tissue damage
- Pathway may not be direct line

2-55

High-energy Penetrating Injuries

FOCUS: **Discuss high-energy injuries and pathways**

How do these weapons differ from handguns and shotguns? How do the wounds differ, internally and externally?

- Greater energy produced
- Greater transfer of energy
- Greater tissue damage
- Pathways may not be direct line
- More extensive exit wounds

2-56

Projectile—Frontal Area

FOCUS: **Discuss the pathophysiology of projectile injuries**

- The larger the frontal area, the greater number of body areas hit and damaged.
- The greater the energy exchange, the larger the cavity created, the greater the exit wound.
- Profile of the projectile determines the area of injury.
- Profile may change shape (mushrooming and/or fragmentation).
- Pathway of the projectile
- Fragmentation of the projectile and/or bone
- Area of coning (cavitation)
- Exit wounds in relation to entrance wounds

2-57

Gunshot Wounds—Cavitation

2-58

FOCUS: **Discuss the difference between entrance and exit wounds and the pathophysiology of gunshot wounds**

Describe the differences between entrance and exit wounds.

- Entrance smaller
- Exit larger due to tissue cavitation

Slide No.	Lecture Content	Notes

2-59   *Tumbling Projectiles*

FOCUS: **Discuss projectile tumbling, related tissue damage, and its pathophysiology**

Some projectiles are designed to tumble. Why?

- Some projectiles are designed to tumble to create greater tissue damage.
- Tumbling can be caused by the rifle design, the projectile design, or by deflection of the projectile.

2-60   *Fragmentation*

FOCUS: **Discuss the pathophysiology of fragmentation**

The shotgun round is the ultimate in fragmentation.

- Fragmentation may be the result of the projectile striking bone structures, not just fragmentation of the projectile.
- Multiple injury sites

2-61   *Considerations for Penetrating Trauma*

FOCUS: **Discuss areas of consideration when treating patients with penetrating trauma**

- Scene safety
- Patient care is the priority!
- Weapon type
- Range at which weapon was fired
- Number of entrance and exit wounds
- Underlying anatomy and track
- Crime scene preservation

Do not allow preservation of a crime scene to prevent you from treating a patient's injuries.

2-62   *Kinematics Summary*

FOCUS: **Emphasize that kinematics must be included and considered whenever assessing a trauma patient**

The cornerstone of assessment is early consideration of kinematics to predict hidden injury.

Patient Assessment

CHAPTER OBJECTIVES

At the completion of this course the student will be able to:

- Explain the importance of the patient assessment process in the overall management of the trauma patient.

- Identify the discrete steps involved in the process of assessing and managing the trauma patient.

- Explain why evaluation of safety, scene, situation, and kinematics are vitally important when performing an assessment.

- Describe the 15-second global evaluation followed by the rest of the primary survey/initial assessment using the A B C D E method.

- Describe the rapid examination skills necessary to evaluate respiration, circulation, and level of consciousness/responsiveness.

- Identify life-threatening conditions that require immediate attention.

- Identify the steps in the secondary survey/focused history and physical examination.

- Understand the importance of the question "Why?"

Slide No.	Lecture Content	Notes

3-1 A *Title Slides*

3-1 B

3-2 *Lesson 3 Objectives*

FOCUS: **Review objectives**

- Define the global evaluation.
- Investigate the use of primary survey.
- Identify life-threatening injuries.
- Define transportation and definitive care.

3-3 *Global Evaluation*

FOCUS: **Discuss scene survey and priorities**

You respond to a two-car collision on a three-lane limited access highway. One car is off the road, and the other has struck a tree. Your unit arrives first.

- What are your priorities?
- What are your SAFETY concerns at this scene?

3-4 *Scene Survey*

FOCUS: **Allow for student discussion of safety concerns**

As you pull up, what concerns you most at this scene?

3-5 *Frontal Impact*

FOCUS: **Allow participants to interact with scenario**

What does this scene tell you about potential injuries?

3-6 *Primary Survey*

FOCUS: **Read and discuss scenario**

Your patient is the 44-year-old male driver of a van that has struck a tree. When you move the air bag, you note a deformed steering wheel. This is your only patient, and he was not wearing a seat belt.

- What steps are you going to take in the assessment of this patient?

3-7 *Primary Survey*

FOCUS: **Discuss findings**

- A—Clear
- B—Rapid, shallow, breath sounds (BS) clear
- C—Rapid, weak radial pulse; delayed capillary refill; no external hemorrhage
- D—Responsive to verbal stimuli, anxious and confused, PEARL
- E—No gross findings. Patient cold, shivering

What do these findings suggest?

Slide No.	Lecture Content	Notes

3-8

Resuscitation

FOCUS: **Life-threatening conditions**

- A—Airway compromise
- B—Inadequate ventilation, oxygenation
- C—Uncontrolled bleeding, tunnel vision
- D—Decreased level of consciousness (LOC), spinal involvement
- E—Hypothermia

Shock or impending shock? When would you manage these conditions?

Treatment

- Rapid extrication, oxygen, a warm environment, transport, IV therapy.

3-9

Primary Survey

FOCUS: **Stress the importance of the primary survey in the critically injured patient**

You may never get past the primary survey if the patient's status is acute.

3-10

Airway

FOCUS: **Examine photo and discuss priorities**

What would your priorities be in caring for this patient?

3-11

Breathing

FOCUS: **Examine photo and discuss priorities**

How would this presentation affect your priorities?

Pitfall: Waiting until the secondary survey to auscultate the lungs

3-12

Circulation

FOCUS: **Examine photo and discuss priorities**

What would your priorities be here?

Pitfall: Not looking for other causes of shock when obvious bleeding is present

3-13

Disability

FOCUS: **Examine photo and discuss priorities**

List your priorities.

Pitfall: Not treating for shock when the patient has an obvious head injury

Slide No.	Lecture Content	Notes

3-14

Expose

FOCUS: **Examine photo and discuss priorities**

What would your priorities be in the care of this patient?

Pitfall: Not exposing a patient and thereby missing a potential life-threat

3-15

Goal

FOCUS: **Discuss the goal of the primary survey**

The goal of the primary survey is to find and treat life-threatening problems.

3-16

Vital Signs

FOCUS: **Review initial assessment**

These vital signs are obtained for you.

- Pulse 120
- Blood pressure (BP) 116/90
- Respiratory rate (RR) 24
- Skin cool and moist

What is the importance of these vital signs? Would you treat the patient?

3-17

Secondary Survey (Focused Exam)

FOCUS: **Review secondary survey**

Findings:

- Negative except for pain on palpation of left lower abdomen. Minor lacerations of left leg. Glasgow Coma Scale (GCS) is 13.

When would you perform the secondary survey?
Do these findings match the mechanism of injury?
Would these findings alter your care?

3-18

Secondary Survey Pitfalls

FOCUS: **Knowing when and how to use the secondary survey**

- Completing a secondary survey on a patient before life threats are managed
- Failing to complete a secondary survey on a critical trauma patient after life threats are managed
- Failing to complete a secondary survey on a stable patient
- Not obtaining the medical history on a trauma patient when possible

Slide No.	Lecture Content	Notes

3-19

Trauma Triage

FOCUS: **Discuss triage methods**

Based on:

- Physiologic criteria
- Anatomic findings
- Mechanism of injury

What are the criteria in your area?

3-20

Transportation of the Critical Patient

FOCUS: **Discuss methods of rapid transport**

Most timely method to get patient to definitive care:

- Ground unit
- Helicopter

3-21

Communication to the Receiving Facility

FOCUS: **Discuss the scope of communication to the receiving facility**

- Medical control
- Patient condition
- Current management
- Potential complications

3-22

Pitfalls

FOCUS: **Review communication pitfalls**

- Late notification—Notification should take place as soon as possible even if a detailed examination has not been completed.
- Failing to react to patient changes—Assess continuously during transport
- Notify receiving hospital of significant changes in patient condition!

3-23

Trauma Score

3-24

FOCUS: **Review the trauma score**

3-25

- Respiratory rate and expansion
- Systolic BP and capillary refill
- GCS (eye opening, verbal response, motor response)
- Total GCS points

3-26

Written Documentation

FOCUS: **Discuss fundamentals of written documentation**

- Well written
- Legal protection
- Case review
- Part of QI

3-27

Patient Assessment Summary

You can't treat what you don't find!

Airway Management and Ventilation

CHAPTER OBJECTIVES

At the completion of this course the student will be able to:

- Identify patients who require airway control.

- Define adequate minute volume and oxygenation and explain their importance as they relate to trauma patients.

- Define reduced perfusion and describe its implications for trauma patients.

- Explain the need for increased oxygenation and tidal volume exchange in trauma patients.

- List methods of manual and mechanical airway management and how to implement them while maintaining in-line cervical spine immobilization.

- List methods of ventilation and how to implement them while maintaining in-line cervical spine immobilization.

- List common errors encountered with bag-valve-mask ventilation.

- List the indications, methods, and common errors of percutaneous transtracheal ventilation, endotracheal intubation, and needle thoracostomy.

- Describe techniques for initial and subsequent assessment of airway and ventilation interventions in trauma patients.

Slide No.	Lecture Content	Notes

4-1 A

4-1 B

Title Slides

4-2

Lesson 4 Objectives

FOCUS: **Review objectives**

- Identify patients in need of airway control.
- Explain the need for increased oxygenation and ventilation in the critical trauma patient.
- Discuss methods of manual and mechanical management of the airway.
- Discuss common errors in ventilation of the trauma patient.

4-3

Airway Assessment and Management

FOCUS: **Help participants understand the keys and tools necessary for proper airway assessment and management; review pitfalls**

Keys:

- Know airway anatomy and physiology.
- Associate symptoms with pathology.
- Know which management tool is most appropriate for each patient.

Tools:

- Observation
- Listening
- Auscultation

Pitfalls:

- Wrong tool for wrong patient condition

4-4

Anatomy—Upper Airway

FOCUS: **Review anatomy and the signs and symptoms specific to upper airway obstruction**

- Noisy respirations = obstructed airway
- Gurgling and snoring indicate that the obstruction is above the larynx.
  - Patients with altered LOC may not have sufficient muscle tone to keep the airway open.
- Stridor and wheezing indicate that the obstruction is at the larynx or below.

4-5

Anatomy—Lower Airway

FOCUS: **Discuss anatomy and function of the lower airways**

- Conduction region—Begins at the trachea and continues to the lungs
- Exchange region—Gas exchange takes place in the alveoli and terminal bronchioles.

Slide No.	Lecture Content	Notes

4-6

Respiratory System

FOCUS: **Discuss function of the respiratory system**

- Ventilation
  - Delivers oxygen to alveoli
- Respiration
  - Exchanges oxygen and carbon dioxide across alveolar-capillary barrier
- Aerobic metabolism

Also discuss the neurologic control of respiration, CO_2 drive, etc.

4-7

Hypoxia

FOCUS: **Hypoxia will cause anaerobic metabolism and acidosis**

What happens if oxygen does not reach the cells of the body?

4-8

Scenario

FOCUS: **Present scenario and allow discussion**

You are doing standby for a football game. After an impressive block, one of the players does not get up. You are called to the field.

What injuries might you suspect, given the mechanism?

4-9

Findings

FOCUS: **What is causing the football player's problems?**

- A—Snoring respirations
- B—Rapid, labored breathing
- C—Strong, rapid radial pulse
- D—Unresponsive
- E—No obvious trauma. Patient still in full uniform, including helmet.

What are your options in managing this patient?

Let students voice their opinions. Remark on the patient's noisy, partially obstructed airway.

4-10

Manual Airway Control

FOCUS: **The importance of controlling the airway**

- Trauma jaw thrust—opens the airway without compromising the C-spine
- Trauma chin lift

Pitfalls:

- Attempting more invasive methods prior to basic technique

The basic technique often works and advanced airway techniques should be delayed until the basic is attempted. In this case, the airway is opened without compromising the C-spine, and as we do so, the football player wakes up.

Slide No.	Lecture Content	Notes

4-11 *Scenario*

FOCUS: **Present the scenario and allow the students to suggest their approach**

You are dispatched to a motorcycle and car collision. Bystanders report that the motorcycle was traveling at about 40 mph when a car pulled in front of the motorcycle. You find the patient laying on the pavement 30 feet away from the collision. His helmet is heavily damaged and has been removed by a bystander.

4-12 *Findings*

FOCUS: **Present findings and discuss**

- A—Snoring respirations, blood in the airway
- B—Respirations are rapid and labored. Breath sounds are coarse, but chest seems intact
- C—Pulse rapid, no obvious external bleeding
- D—Responsive to painful stimuli
- E—No major external trauma noted, but patient is cyanotic.

What problems does this patient have?

4-13 *Discussion*

FOCUS: **Discuss with students**

- Impact may have produced severe injury.
- Respiratory noise always means obstruction.
- Rapid breathing and cyanosis indicate poor exchange, causing hypoxia and acidosis.
- Altered LOC can impair the patient's ability to manage the airway.

4-14 *Mechanical Methods*

4-15 FOCUS: **Discuss each device and its uses**

- Suctioning
- Oropharyngeal airway (OPA)
- Nasopharyngeal airway (NPA)
- Multi-lumen airways (Combitube®/PtL®)
- Laryngeal mask airways (LMA)
- Orotracheal intubation
- Nasotracheal intubation
- Transtracheal ventilation

Which method would you choose to manage this patient?

Slide No.	Lecture Content	Notes

4-16   *Suctioning*

FOCUS: **Discuss preferences with suction: hard, large-bore (i.e., rigid suction) catheters**

- Used to remove secretions from the airway

Pitfalls:

- Causes or worsens hypoxia

4-17   *Oropharyngeal Airway (OPA)*

FOCUS: **Discuss the use of oral airways**

- Not indicated if gag reflex present
- Best used temporarily
- Does not protect the trachea

4-18   *Nasopharyngeal Airway (NPA)*

FOCUS: **Discuss the use of nasopharyngeal airways**

- When would you use this device?
- What are its limitations?

4-19   *Multi-lumen Airways*

FOCUS: **Describe the use of multi-lumen airways**

- How do they work?
- What are the indications for use?
- What are the contraindications for use?

4-20   *Laryngeal Mask Airway (LMA)*

FOCUS: **Present as information only; the LMA is not widely available or advocated in the United States**

Inflatable silicone ring attached diagonally to a silicone tube. Used during prehospital stage in Europe.
  Advantages:

- Designed for blind insertion
- Only minimally stimulating to the upper airway
- Available in a range of sizes
- Reusable

Note: Indicated for this patient

4-21   *Intubation with In-line Stabilization*

4-22   FOCUS: **The indications and techniques that will be demontrated in the skill station**

- What are the indications for oral endotracheal tube placement?
- When do we use the in-line technique?
  Pitfalls:

- Improper tube placement
- Hypoxia from improper technique

Slide No.	Lecture Content	Notes

4-23

Nasotracheal Intubation

FOCUS: **The indications, techniques, and concerns for nasotracheal intubation**

When would you perform nasotracheal intubation?
　Pitfalls:

- Improper tube placement
- Hypoxia from improper technique
- Bleeding

4-24

Transtracheal Ventilation

4-25

FOCUS: **The indications for transtracheal ventilation and the techniques that will be demonstrated in the skill station**

Indications:

- Last resort
- Upper airway obstruction
- Can support CO_2 for 20 to 30 minutes

What are the limitations?

- Does not isolate the trachea

4-26

Airway Management

FOCUS: **Stress the importance of adequately assessing and stabilizing the airway**

Pitfalls:

- Failure to adequately control the airway in a patient with a prolonged alteration of the LOC.
- Inaccurately assessing the airway to determine proper placement of the device.

4-27

Oxygen

FOCUS: **Stress the importance of oxygen**

- Once the airway is controlled, supplemental oxygen must be administered.
- Goal is to choose a device that will deliver an FiO_2 of at least .85.

4-28

Oxygen

FOCUS: **Pitfalls of oxygenation**

Pitfall: Thinking that an FiO_2 will correct a minute ventilation problem.

Slide No.	Lecture Content	Notes

4-29

Lung Volumes

FOCUS: **Present normal lung volumes**

Tidal volume (Vt)

- Normal 500 cc

Dead space

- 150 cc

Minute volume (MV)

- MV = Tidal volume × Respiratory rate
- Normal 6,500 to 7,500 ml air

4-30

Minute Volume

FOCUS: **Describe minute volume**

Patient breathing

- Vt = 600 cc
- RR = 12
- Minute volume = 7,200 cc

Patient breathing

- Vt = 200 cc
- RR = 20
- Minute volume = 4,000 cc

4-31

Minute Volume Rates

FOCUS: **Reinforce that inadequate respirations will severely reduce minute volume and result in hypoxia**

Minute volume is usually inadequate in patients who breathe *slower* than 10 to 12 bpm or *faster* than 28 to 30 bpm.

4-32

Scenario

FOCUS: **Present scenario and allow discussion**

You are dispatched to a ski racer who has hit a tree at the bottom of a trail. A friend who was skiing with him tells you he was traveling very fast and lost control, hitting the tree at full speed.

4-33

Findings

FOCUS: **Present findings and discuss**

- A—Noisy airway contains blood, broken teeth
- B—Respiratory rate is 38, shallow. Breathing appears to be painful. Breath sounds (BS) are clear.
- C—Weak radial pulse of about 120
- D—Responsive to painful stimuli
- E—Deformity to right knee, helmet damage

Do you think the minute volume is adequate? What are the possible causes of the problem?

Slide No.	Lecture Content	Notes

4-34 *Ventilation*

FOCUS: **Discuss the purpose of ventilation and devices for administering ventilation**

- To improve minute volume and oxygenation
- Bag-valve-mask
- Oxygen-powered demand valves
- Transport ventilators

4-35 *Bag-valve-masks (BVM)*

FOCUS: **Describe the proper techniques for best efficiency with BVM to be demonstrated in skill station**

- Minimum of 800 cc per breath
- 95% to 100% oxygen
- May require two or three rescuers
- Maintain alignment of C-spine

4-36 *Oxygen-Powered Demand Valves*

FOCUS: **Discuss the advantages and disadvantages of oxygen-powered demand valves**

Positive:
- Easy to make a seal and ventilate by a single rescuer

Negatives:
- Hyperinflation
- Hypoinflation
- No feel for compliance
- Promotes gastric distention

4-37 *Transport Ventilators*

FOCUS: **Highly specialized equipment usually found on specialty vehicles and aeromed units**

- Delivered volume remains constant.
- Pressure changes with compliance.
- Ability to maintain PEEP
- Hands-free operation
- Alarms

4-38 *Airway Management Summary*

FOCUS: **Stress the importance of adequate and timely assessment and stabilization of the airway**

Providing a patent airway and oxygenation early for the trauma patient improves outcome.

Thoracic Trauma

CHAPTER OBJECTIVES

At the completion of this course the student will be able to:

- Identify the general anatomy of the chest.

- Describe the normal anatomy and physiology neccessary for adequate ventilation.

- Define the associated pathology and pathophysiology pertinent to ventilation and circulation in the thorax.

- List the basic diagnostic signs and treatment of the following:
  a. rib fractures
  b. flail chest
  c. pulmonary contusion
  d. pneumothorax (open and closed)
  e. tension pneumothorax and hemothorax
  f. myocardial contusion
  g. pericardial tamponade
  h. aortic, tracheal, and bronchial rupture
  i. traumatic asphyxiation
  j. diaphragmatic rupture

- Define the relationship of kinematics to thoracic trauma.

- Identify the need for rapid stabilization and transportation to the hospital.

Slide No.	Lecture Content	Notes

5-1 A   *Title Slides*

5-1 B

5-2   *Lesson 5 Objectives*

FOCUS: **Review objectives**

- Review the anatomy of the chest.
- Discuss the mechanics of breathing.
- Detail the assessment process.
- Cover the management of:
  - Rib fractures
  - Flail chest
  - Pulmonary contusion
  - Pneumothorax
  - Tension pneumothorax
  - Myocardial contusion
  - Pericardial tamponade
  - Aortic rupture
  - Traumatic asphyxia

5-3   *Introduction*

FOCUS: **Early field interventions for chest injuries can save lives**

- Chest injuries are the second leading cause of trauma deaths each year.
- Chest injuries often go unrecognized.
- Missed injuries result in inadequate ventilation, hypoxia, and hypercarbia.
- Our goal is to find these injuries early and treat them aggressively.

Injuries cause alterations in gas exchange via several mechanisms: injuries such as rib fractures, flail chest, and pneumothorax disturb respiratory mechanics and injuries such as a pulmonary contusion alter gas exchange.

   Injuries cause alterations in blood flow: an aortic rupture may cause hypovolemia, tension pneumothorax or pericardial tamponade impair blood return to the heart, and myocardial contusion or pericardial tamponade impair cardiac output.

5-4   *Anatomy*

FOCUS: **It is important to understand the anatomy, in order to understand the potential injuries given a particular mechanism of injury**

Identify these structures in the thorax:

- Trachea
- Bronchi
- Lobes of the lungs
- Heart
- Aorta
- Vena cava
- Esophagus

Slide No.	Lecture Content	Notes

5-5

Physiology

FOCUS: **Understand the mechanics of inspiration and expiration**

- What happens to the chest on inspiration and expiration?
- How does the air move into and out of the chest?

Inspiration requires the voluntary contraction of the diaphragm and the intercostal muscles, resulting in decreased intrathoracic pressure and air flow into the lungs. Expiration is a passive function, when the same muscles relax, causing a rise in intrathoracic pressure and gas flow out of the lungs.

5-6

Gas Exchange in the Lungs

FOCUS: **Respiration is controlled by the exchange of O_2 and CO_2**

5-7

Neurochemical Control

FOCUS: **Understand the body's major respiratory center and its effect on the respiratory rate**

The respiratory control center is located in the brain stem. It reacts to changes in the concentration of CO_2 in the blood.

- What happens when the CO_2 level increases?
- What happens to the CO_2 level if the patient's ventilation decreases?
- Name some traumatic conditions that would increase the CO_2 level in the blood.

When CO_2 increases, the respiratory center senses the change and stimulates a higher respiratory rate to eliminate the excess carbon dioxide.

If the patient hypoventilates, the arterial CO_2 increases, and the patient becomes acidotic.

Any condition that alters the ability to properly ventilate and get rid of CO_2 (i.e., rib fractures), impairs the passage of gases across the capillary/alveoli barrier (pulmonary contusion), or causes shock (increases CO_2 production).

5-8

Assessment of Chest Trauma

FOCUS: **Primary survey should identify most life-threatening chest injuries that require field intervention**

- The initial assessment should serve to detect most major chest injuries.
- The kinematics of the event will point to most major chest trauma.
- Pain from chest trauma tends to be provoked by deep inspiration and/or firm palpation.

Slide No.	Lecture Content	Notes

5-9   *Assessment of Chest Trauma*

FOCUS: **Assessment of the chest requires careful examination techniques to pick up the sometimes subtle findings of chest injuries**

Observation
- What are we looking for?

Palpation
- Why are we feeling the chest?

Auscultation
- What are we listening for in the chest?

Observe for asymmetric chest wall expansion, respiratory splinting, or paradoxical motion. Palpate for deformities and crepitus. Listen for presence, quality, and nature of breath sounds in both lung fields.

5-10   *Chest Trauma*

FOCUS: **Many different mechanisms of injury may cause thoracic injuries**

Chest trauma falls into two categories, based on mechanism of injury.
- Penetrating
- Blunt

Can you name some mechanisms of injury for each?
- Penetrating: Gunshot wounds, stab wounds
- Blunt: Motor vehicle crashes, assault with a blunt instrument, falls

5-11   *Scenario*

FOCUS: **Blunt mechanism for chest injury**

You are responding to a call to the police station where a 19-year-old male patient is complaining of chest pain. Upon arrival you learn that your patient was kicked in the chest during a fight.
- What injuries does the mechanism suggest?

Rib fractures, flail chest, pulmonary contusion, pneumothorax

5-12   *Findings*

FOCUS: **Using kinematics and the primary survey, injuries are anticipated and identified**
- A—Clear
- B—Left-sided chest pain during inspiration; BS equal
- C—Normal pulse, no external bleeding
- D—Alert and oriented × 3
- Vitals: Pulse 98, RR 26, BP 122/74

Slide No.	Lecture Content	Notes

Given the findings, what injuries can you rule out? How should this patient be managed?

Major, immediately life-threatening injuries are probably not present. Breath sounds are equal, so pneumothorax is unlikely. Rib fractures are likely, and an underlying pulmonary contusion is possible. Oxygen, immobilization, and transport to a hospital should be provided.

5-13

Scenario

FOCUS: **Falls from significant heights may cause serious injuries**

You are called to a farm for a worker who has fallen from a hayloft and impaled himself on a post. On arrival, you see him lying on the ground in obvious respiratory distress. The scene appears safe.

- What injuries would you suspect?

5-14

Findings

FOCUS: **Identify injuries during the primary and secondary surveys**

- A—Clear
- B—Rapid, paradoxical movement of the right chest, BS decreased on that side
- C—Rapid radial pulse
- D—Alert, oriented × 3
- Vitals: Pulse 118, RR 38, BP 106/80

Given the findings, what injuries do you suspect? How should this patient be managed?

Deceleration type injuries—blunt injuries to thorax from impact with ground or other obstacles

Paradoxical chest wall motion: flail chest. Decreased breath sounds on right: pneumothorax. Must be aware of potential for deceleration injury: ruptured aorta. Management: oxygen, immobilization, rapid transport to appropriate facility. Monitor closely for deterioration: tension pneumothorax, hypoventilation, hypovolemia.

5-15

Scenario

FOCUS: **Penetrating trauma—consider ballistics and wounding potential of the particular weapon**

You respond to the aid of a 16-year-old male gunshot victim. Police inform you that the weapon was a .22-caliber handgun.

- What do you know about .22-caliber bullets?

Handgun, penetrating trauma, medium velocity weapon, zone of injury, temporary and permanent cavitation.

Slide No.	Lecture Content	Notes

5-16

Findings

FOCUS: **Penetrating chest trauma carries the potential of life-threatening injuries**

- A—Clear
- B—Fast, BS diminished on right. Entrance wound noted in right anterior chest wall
- C—Pulse rapid, no external bleeding noted
- D—Alert, oriented × 3
- Vitals: Pulse 114, RR 32, BP 108/78

What is your major concern for this patient?

Massive intrathoracic hemorrhage, tension pneumothorax, cardiac injury with tamponade. Oxygen, close monitoring, rapid transport to appropriate facility, needle thoracostomy if necessary.

5-17

Scenario

FOCUS: **Falling from a significant height may cause lethal injuries; index of suspicion**

You respond to an industrial incident where a 48-year-old male has fallen 15 feet from some scaffolding and landed on some equipment. On your arrival you find him complaining of chest pain and difficulty breathing.

5-18

Findings

FOCUS: **Perform primary survey to identify life-threatening injuries and treat as they are found**

- A—Clear
- B—Rapid, shallow; speaking in 2 to 3 word bursts, BS absent on left, pain on palpation of left chest. JVD noted.
- C—Rapid weak pulse, no external bleeding noted
- D—Alert, oriented × 3. PEARL

What are this patient's problems? What are your treatment priorities?

Probable tension pneumothorax. Must keep in mind possibility of blunt cardiac injury with tamponade. Oxygen, immobilization, needle thoracostomy, rapid transport to appropriate facility.

5-19

Tension vs. Simple Pneumothorax

FOCUS: **Differentiation between simple and tension pneumothorax may not always be simple; patient's physiologic stability often is the key factor**

Simple pneumothorax:

- Decreased or absent BS
- Mechanism of injury

Slide No.	Lecture Content	Notes

Tension pneumothorax:

- Decreased or absent BS
- Mechanism of injury
- Hemodynamic compromise

Inequality of breath sounds is often difficult to determine in the field. JVD may not be present in the hypovolemic patient. Tracheal deviation is easy to see on a chest X ray, but not on a real patient. The key is high index of suspicion with a hemodynamically unstable patient.

5-20

Scenario

FOCUS: **High speed impact means high energy trauma. Rapid deceleration injuries are probable**

Your patient is a 37-year-old female who was involved in a head-on MVC. Looking at the car, you surmise that this was a high-energy impact. The patient has been extricated on your arrival.

5-21

Findings

FOCUS: **Blunt chest trauma may cause injuries to the heart and great vessels**

- A—Clear
- B—RR slightly elevated, BS clear, bruising over sternum
- C—Pulse irregular, no external bleeding
- D—Alert, oriented × 3, PEARL
- Vitals: Pulse 88 and irregular, RR 20, BP 132/80

What is this patient's problem? How would you treat her?

Myocardial contusion may be present, with the potential for tamponade. Aortic rupture with rapid deceleration must be kept in mind. Oxygen, immobilization, close monitoring, dysrhythmia therapy for hemodynamically significant rhythms, and rapid transport to an appropriate facility are necessary.

5-22

Myocardial Compression Injuries

FOCUS: **Significant myocardial contusion is rare, but when present, it may be catastrophic**

There are three distinct injury patterns that can occur with compression of the chest:

- Electrical conduction disturbance
- Myocardial contusion
- Myocardial rupture

Slide No.	Lecture Content	Notes

5-23

Discussion

FOCUS: **Rare injury, but must be aware of possibility and intervene as necessary**

- May decrease cardiac output
- May mimic a myocardial infarction
- Treatment:
  - Oxygen
  - Rapid transport
  - Cardiac monitor (ALS intervention)
  - Drugs (ALS intervention)

5-24

Myocardial Rupture/Cardiac Tamponade/Traumatic Asphyxia

FOCUS: **Traumatic cardiac tamponade is a rapidly fatal condition**

- Pressures as high as 800 mm Hg can develop in the heart and great vessels when the sternum is compressed.
- Rupture of the myocardium fills the fibrous sac that surrounds the heart with blood, eventually tamponading the heart.
- Name the signs and symptoms of cardiac tamponade.

Muffled heart sounds (essentially impossible to discern in the field). Narrowed pulse pressure (essentially impossible to measure in the field). JVD (may be absent in the hypovolemic trauma patient). Probably the most reliable symptom in the awake patient is the sense of impending doom.

5-25

Thoracic Trauma Summary

FOCUS: **Stress the connection between thoracic trauma and oxygenation of blood and the need for timely treatment**

Because the thoracic cavity contains the vital organs that oxygenate and distribute blood to the rest of the body, timely recognition and treatment of chest injuries result in better patient outcomes.

LESSON 6

Shock and Fluid Resuscitation

CHAPTER OBJECTIVES

At the completion of this course the student will be able to:

- Define perfusion, hypoperfusion, hypoxia, hypovolemia, normovolemia, hypervolemia, and hypotension.

- Define the pathophysiology of shock, including the three phases of shock and their progression.

- List the signs and symptoms of each phase of shock.

- Explain the proper use of the pneumatic antishock garment.

- List the indications for intravenous fluid replacement.

- Identify the need for rapid transport when confronted with continuing hypoperfusion.

- Demonstrate an understanding for the limits and short-term benefits of crystalloid fluid replacement and pneumatic antishock garment usage.

- Demonstrate an understanding of the need for blood replacement and hemorrhage control as the definitive care for blood loss.

- Explain why severe internal hemorrhage, even if temporarily controlled with a pressure dressing, needs to have direct surgical control in the operating room without delay.

Slide No.	Lecture Content	Notes

6-1 A

6-1 B

Title Slides

6-2

Lesson 6 Objectives

FOCUS: **Review objectives**

- Correlate perfusion, hypoperfusion, hypoxia, hypovolemia, and hypotension to the signs and symptoms of shock.
- Differentiate between early and late signs of shock.
- Describe the pathophysiologic changes of shock.
- Identify the management of shock, including conservation of heat, fluid replacement, and the pneumatic antishock garment.

6-3

Shock

FOCUS: **Review definition, elicit comments**

A rude unhinging of the machinery of life

Samuel Gross, 1852

6-4

Shock Redefined

FOCUS: **Definition of shock emphasis should be on perfusion not BP**

Lack of end-tissue perfusion

  Pitfall:

- Defining shock as decreased blood pressure

6-5

Scenario

FOCUS: **This scenario will serve as the reference point for anatomy and pathophysiology of shock for the remainder of the lecture**

You are caring for the sole victim of a motorcycle crash. He is lying on the ground next to his motorcycle. The scene appears safe.

6-6

Findings

FOCUS: **Review the scenario as an example of the classic patient in shock**

- A—Open, clear
- B—RR fast, BS clear, bruising noted over sternum, no other chest deformity
- C—Radial pulse weak and rapid
- D—PEARL; anxious and confused; normal movement and sensation
- E—No deformity noted, skin cool and diaphoretic

Slide No.	Lecture Content	Notes

6-7 *Discussion*

FOCUS: **Encourage students to interact**

- Is this patient in shock?
- Why?
- What is the patient's real problem?

The patient is in shock. Students should voice signs and symptoms. The real problem is inadequate tissue perfusion.

6-8 *Cell Perfusion*

FOCUS: **Remind students that this patient is undergoing anaerobic metabolism**

- Aerobic metabolism requires adequate oxygenation.
- Cells require oxygen and sugar to produce energy and carbon dioxide.

Is the patient in the scenario adequately perfusing his cells?

6-9 *Anaerobic Metabolism*

FOCUS: **Remind students that anaerobic metabolism is inefficient and produces acid**

Inadequate oxygenation for metabolism

By-products:

- Less energy
- More acid
- Potassium

6-10 *Cellular Death*

FOCUS: **Remind students that cell death leads to organism death without early intervention**

Pitfall:

- If cellular death is not prevented, organism death will follow.

6-11 *Staged Death*

FOCUS: **Death can occur rapidly or be delayed. Signs and symptoms correlate with the stage of shock.**

Organism death:

- May be quick—prior to EMS
- May be prolonged—2 to 3 weeks later

Occurs in stages:

- Stages occur as the body tries to compensate.
- We see the stages through signs and symptoms.

Slide No.	Lecture Content	Notes

6-12

Prevent Cellular Death

FOCUS: **Review the keys to preventing cellular death; early intervention is the primary key**

- Recognize shock early.
- Restore cellular perfusion.
- Restore aerobic metabolism.

Pitfall:

- Waiting until it is too late to restore perfusion to cells

6-13

Early Recognition

FOCUS: **Review the signs and symptoms commonly associated with compensated and uncompensated shock**

6-14

Early vs. Late

FOCUS: **Review the early signs of shock vs. the late signs of shock**

- What are the earliest signs of shock?
- What is a late sign of shock?

6-15

Restore Cellular Perfusion

FOCUS: **Review the concept that balances must be maintained to maintain adequate perfusion**

- Maintain *chemical* balance
- Maintain *fluid* balance

6-16

Chemical Balance

FOCUS: **What occurs when O_2 and CO_2 levels are altered?**

Decrease in oxygen

- Detected by chemical receptors in the carotid arteries and in the arch of the aorta
- Respirations increase in rate and depth

Rise in acidity

- Buffer system converts the acid to CO_2 and water.
- Medulla senses increased CO_2.
- Respirations increase and CO_2 is blown off.

6-17

Chemical Balance

FOCUS: **What occurs when O_2 and CO_2 levels are altered?**

- Key: Increase in respiratory rate is an early sign of shock.
- What signs or symptoms indicate that the patient's body is trying to restore its chemical balance?
- What steps could you take to help the body restore balance and aerobic metabolism?

Slide No.	Lecture Content	Notes

6-18

Fluid Decrease

FOCUS: **The neurologic response to fluid decreases**

6-19

Fluid Decrease

FOCUS: **Review the hormonal response to fluid decreases**

Hormonal response:

- Various hormones are released, causing vasoconstriction and fluid retention.

Compensation:

- Blood vessels constrict.
- Heart increases strength and rate.
- Fluid is retained.

6-20

Fluid Decrease

FOCUS: **Correlate patient signs and symptoms to compensatory mechanisms and review what EMS providers can do to improve compensation**

- In the scenario, which signs suggest that the patient's body was trying to restore its fluid balance?
- Is the patient compensating well? Why?
- What steps could you take to help the body restore balance?

Emphasize that this patient is not compensating well. The patient needs definitive care and fluid resuscitation.

6-21

The Fick Principle

FOCUS: **Discuss the Fick principle**

- Defines what is necessary to achieve end tissue perfusion
  - On-loading oxygen to the RBCs
  - Delivering the RBCs to the tissue
  - Off-loading oxygen to the tissue
- As part of the process, patient must have an adequate number of RBCs to transport oxygen.

6-22

Scenario

FOCUS: **Correlate patient to Fick principle and compensation**

You are responding to a patient who has fallen from a 40-foot cliff while rock climbing. He is awake. He tells you he can't move his legs and has no feeling below his waist. Vital signs: pulse 119, RR 20, and BP 104/72.

- How does the Fick principle apply here?
- How well is this patient compensating?

He may not have enough RBCs due to possible hemorrhage. He is compensating at this time—elevated pulse rate.

Slide No.	Lecture Content	Notes

6-23

Scenario

FOCUS: **Correlate patient to Fick principle and compensation**

You are called to the scene of a house fire, where firefighters have just removed one patient. He is unresponsive. His vital signs are pulse 102, RR 6, and BP 104/76.

- How does the Fick principle apply here?
- How well is this patient compensating?

Trouble on-loading due to respiratory and enclosed space fire. Trouble off-loading due to CO from fire. Not compensating well.

6-24

Scenario

FOCUS: **Correlate patient to Fick principle and compensation**

You respond to the scene where a skier has struck a tree at high speed. Examination reveals pain on palpation of the right lateral chest, absent breath sounds on the right, and labored breathing. Vital signs: pulse 142, RR 40, BP 88/70.

- How does the Fick principle apply here?
- How well is this patient compensating?

Not on-loading due to lung injury. Not delivering RBCs to tissue due to BP. May not have enough RBCs due to possible hemorrhage. May not be off-loading due to hypothermia. Not compensating well.

6-25

Scenario

FOCUS: **Correlate patient to Fick principle and compensation**

You are dispatched to a motor vehicle crash. On arrival you find a 47-year-old male driver still in the vehicle. There are 10 to 15 inches of intrusion to the front of the vehicle. The patient is unresponsive as you approach.

6-26

Findings

FOCUS: **Correlate patient to Fick principle and compensation**

- A—Blood and vomitus in airway
- B—Slow and labored. BS absent on left
- C—No palpable radial pulse; cool wet skin; no external bleeding
- D—Pupils equal but reacting slowly
- E—Obvious fracture of left femur

How does the Fick principle apply here?
How well is this patient compensating?

   Not on-loading due to lung injury. Not delivering RBCs to tissue due to decreased BP. May not have enough RBCs due to possible hemorrhage. Not compensating well—decompensating quickly.

6-27

Shock Summary

Shock is staged death—catch it in the first act!

Abdominal Trauma and Trauma in the Pregnant Patient

CHAPTER OBJECTIVES

At the completion of this course the student will be able to:

- Identify the general anatomy of the abdomen.

- Define the physiology and pathophysiology of blunt and penetrating injury to the abdomen.

- Identify the importance of maintaining a high index of suspicion for abdominal trauma.

- List the focused and detailed assessment findings of intra-abdominal bleeding.

- Define the relationship of kinematics to abdominal trauma.

- Explain the importance of abdominal and pelvic hemorrhage control by direct compression using the pneumatic antishock garment along with limitations of its use in certain patients and the later stages of pregnancy.

- Identify the need for rapid intervention and rapid transport when appropriate.

- Identify the anatomic and physiologic changes that occur in pregnancy.

- Identify the proper position for transport of the pregnant trauma patient.

- Understand the physiology of the two lives involved in the management of the pregnant patient.

Slide No.	Lecture Content	Notes

7-1 A *Title Slides*

7-1 B

7-2 *Abdominal Trauma*

7-3 *Lesson 7 Objectives (Abdominal Trauma)*
FOCUS: **Review objectives**
- Associate blunt and penetrating abdominal trauma with anatomy, physiology, and pathophysiology.
- Use mechanism of injury and index of suspicion when assessing, treating, and prioritizing abdominal trauma.
- Identify the appropriate assessment and management of abdominal trauma and the limitations of each.

7-4 *Abdominal Trauma*
FOCUS: **Importance of abdominal trauma**
- Abdominal trauma often goes unrecognized.
- Second leading cause of trauma death.
- Extent of damage difficult to determine.
- Massive blood loss can lead to shock and death.

7-5 *Abdominal Assessment*
FOCUS: **Keys and tools for abdominal assessment**
Keys:
- Anatomy—to identify structures that may be damaged
- Mechanism
- Index of suspicion

Tools:
- Observation for wounds, guarding, positioning
- Palpation for rigidity, tenderness, and masses

Pitfall: Auscultation is a tool, but it is not recommended in the prehospital setting.

7-6 *Penetrating Trauma*
FOCUS: **External appearance of penetrating trauma**
Patient is a victim of multiple gunshot wounds to the abdomen.

Pitfall: Injury significance missed due to lack of attention to kinematics

7-7 *Anatomy*
FOCUS: **Correlating the underlying or associated injuries with the external wounds**
How can you use anatomy to evaluate this patient?
- Organ location
- Solid vs. hollow

Slide No.	Lecture Content	Notes

- Bleeding vs. peritonitis
- Associated chest injury

Use the wound location to determine structures involved. Both solid and hollow organs may be injured. The major immediate concern is hemorrhage. Peritonitis is a concern but is usually a later finding. Due to close proximity, possible trajectory, and cavitation, associated chest injury may be present. Is this patient potentially critical? Yes, major organ involvement, hemorrhage, and chest injury are possible.

7-8

Frontal Impact

FOCUS: **Mechanism; visual picture of speed, damage, and impact type**

You are dispatched to a one-vehicle MVC with one occupant. The scene is safe.

7-9

Blunt Trauma

FOCUS: **Type of patient involved with this type of MVC**

Your patient is the victim of an MVC. Her van struck a pole head on and there is moderate damage to the van. She was wearing a seat belt, and it was positioned over the soft part of her abdomen.

- A—Airway clear
- B—Breathing rapid and shallow
- C—Skin cool and diaphoretic, weak radials, rapid heart rate
- D—Confused and anxious
- E—Bruising to left clavicle area and abdomen above iliac crest. Abdomen is soft and nontender.

7-10

Mechanism of Injury

FOCUS: **Correlating severity with visual cues of damage during vehicle impact, body impact, and organ impact**

Is the patient in this scenario critical or noncritical?

- What was the speed?
  - 40 to 50 mph, speed was enough to cause moderate front-end damage to the vehicle
- What type of impact occurred?
  - Frontal, so we need to think of compression and deceleration effects on the internal organs liver, spleen, bowel, aorta
- What do you see inside the car?
  - Seat belt over the soft part of abdomen.
- What internal organs might be involved?
  - Location of the seat belt and seat belt bruise indicate potential for internal organs to be compressed against spinal column—duodenum, large and small bowel, aorta. Deceleration injuries to liver, kidneys, and spleen.
- Are there signs and symptoms of shock?
  - Rapid and shallow breathing, cool and diaphoretic skin, and confusion and anxiousness all indicate early shock.

Slide No.	Lecture Content	Notes

7-11

Index of Suspicion

FOCUS: **List of indicators for index of suspicion**

Reliable indicators for index of suspicion:

- Mechanism of injury
- Unexplained indicators of shock
- Outward signs of trauma
- Level of shock greater than explained by other injuries

7-12

Index of Suspicion Pitfalls

FOCUS: **Traumatic events where abdominal injuries do not present with expected signs and symptoms**

- Blood in the abdomen may not always cause abdominal pain or tenderness.
- Retroperitoneal injuries are initially asymptomatic.

7-13

Mechanism of Injury

FOCUS: **Correlating index of suspicion to mechanism and assessment findings to severity**

Which of these should increase your index of suspicion that this patient might be seriously injured?

- A—Airway clear
- B—Breathing—18 breaths per minute, labored; lungs clear and equal
- C—Skin cool and dry, radial pulse 110
- D—Anxious, intoxicated
- E—Bruising to right thorax and hip, abdomen soft, nontender

Clear airway is not a factor. Slightly increased respiratory rate may indicate early shock; no immediate indication of life-threatening chest injury. Cool and diaphoretic, slight tachycardia—indicators of early shock. Anxious—early shock indicator; intoxicated—may mask symptoms of pain. Bruising indicates potential underlying injuries; nontender abdomen does not rule out blood in the abdomen, and retroperitoneal injuries are initially asymptomatic. All of these factors should increase your index of suspicion.

7-14

Other Assessment Findings

FOCUS: **Structures retroperitoneal and lack of expected abdominal complaints**

You respond to a patient involved in a fight. He has been hit in the back and flanked with a heavy piece of pipe. He has no complaints of abdominal pain. The scene is safe.

- Injuries to the back may involve retroperitoneal structures like the kidneys, aorta, and vena cava.
- They often present with back pain rather than expected abdominal complaints and findings.

Slide No.	Lecture Content	Notes

7-15 *Evisceration and Impaled Objects*

FOCUS: **Treatment**

You respond to a patient stabbed in the abdomen. A piece of bowel is eviscerated and the knife is still impaled. How would you manage this patient?

- Cover the exposed bowel with moist sterile dressings. Why?
- Stabilize the knife in place. Do not remove impaled objects.
- Pneumatic antishock garment (PASG) contraindicated.

7-16 *Pelvic Fractures*

FOCUS: **Bleeding and PASG**

You respond to a rollover MVC. The patient's pelvis was crushed when the small tractor he was driving rolled over.

- What is significant about this injury?
  - Blood loss is usually significant and occurs retroperitoneal.
- Can PASG be used to stabilize fractures and control bleeding?

7-17 *Abdominal Trauma Management*

FOCUS: **The general management of abdominal trauma**

- Rapid evaluation
  - Rapid assessment to determine severity based on mechanism of injury and index of suspicion
- Shock therapy
  - To include high flow oxygenation
- PASG
  - If indicated according to local protocol
- Rapid transport to the appropriate facility with surgical intervention immediately available
  - Surgical intervention must be immediately available
- IV therapy en route
  - Start IVs en route to the hospital

7-18 *Trauma in Pregnancy*

7-19 *Lesson 7 Objectives (Trauma in Pregnancy)*

FOCUS: **Review of objectives**

- Identify the implications of the anatomic and physiologic changes of pregnancy for the trauma patient.
- Identify the appropriate assessment, management, and priorities for the pregnant trauma patient.

7-20 *Normal Changes with Pregnancy*

FOCUS: **Review the normal changes that occur during pregnancy and discuss picture of pregnant patient**

- Increased heart rate of 15 to 20 beats/min
- Decreased blood pressure
- Increased cardiac output
- Increased blood volume

Slide No.	Lecture Content	Notes

7-21

Normal Pregnancy Changes

FOCUS: **Review the normal changes that occur during pregnancy and discuss picture showing anatomy of pregnancy**

- Increased size of uterus
- Decreased peristalsis
- Loosening of ligaments

7-22

Trauma in Pregnancy

FOCUS: **Scenario to associate mechanism with priorities**

You respond to the scene of a car that struck a guardrail at 60 mph and is resting upright in a ditch. The patient is a 24-year-old female who is 26 weeks (6.5 months) pregnant. There is moderate damage to the car. She was wearing a seat belt.

Given the mechanism, what are the priorities for this patient?

- Mechanism: 60 mph—high speed
- Frontal impact: May have struck steering wheel with abdomen so chance of abruptio placentae or other bleeding associated with pregnant uterus
- Increased chance for spinal involvement due to loose ligaments
- Seat belt may have caused internal damage to pregnant uterus due to high speed

7-23

Findings

FOCUS: **Scenario to differentiate between normal pregnancy changes and shock**

- A—Clear
- B—Breathing—20 breaths per minute, slightly labored and shallow; lungs clear
- C—Pulse 114, skin warm and dry
- D—Anxious
- E—No obvious injury noted
- Vitals: BP 92/56

Are these changes due to trauma or pregnancy?

Monitor for vomiting as her stomach is probably full. The slightly labored and shallow breathing is probably not due to pregnancy. Respiratory rate is usually normal in pregnant women, so look for another cause. BP is decreased. These are normal findings in the second trimester, but shock may also be possible since she can lose up to 35% of her blood volume before showing signs and symptoms of hemorrhage. Anxiety may be due to incident, but it is also an early sign of shock. The mechanism and the ability for a pregnant patient to mask the signs and symptoms of shock dictate that this patient must be treated as serious and monitored for changes.

Slide No.	Lecture Content	Notes

7-24

The Baby

FOCUS: **Reminder: resuscitation has to focus on the mother**

Resuscitation of the BABY depends on aggressive resuscitation of the mother. Why?

   The mother treats the uterus and baby as a peripheral structure and will shunt blood away from the uterus in times of shock. With her increased blood volume, the mother may stay perfused while the baby is not. The focus is to maintain the mother's perfusion, and she will perfuse the baby. Once again index of suspicion is key to both patients surviving.

7-25

Trauma in Pregnancy

FOCUS: **Scenario illustrating signs and symptoms of supine hypotension**

You are dispatched to the scene of a 23-year-old female who is 32 weeks pregnant. She was pushed down a flight of stairs and is found lying on her back.

- A—Clear
- B—Breathing—18 breaths per minute, slightly labored, clear breath sounds.
- C—Very weak radial pulse of 120, no external hemorrhage
- D—Responsive to verbal stimuli
- E—Contusion to right temporal region of head
- Vitals: BP is 86/54; secondary survey is negative except for head contusion

7-26

Discussion

FOCUS: **Treatment of supine hypotension, consider eclampsia**

- How would you manage this patient?
- What condition mimics a head injury?

A possible cause of hypotension is position. Supine hypotension occurs when a pregnant female lies on her back causing the uterus to rest on the vena cava. This decreases the blood return to the heart and drops the cardiac output. This symptom can be relieved by positioning the patient on her left side. If she needs to be immobilized to a backboard, place her on the board and then tilt the spine board 10 to 15 degrees to her left using blanket or towel rolls.

   Eclamptic patients may present with decreased level of consciousness and seizure activity.

Pitfall:

- Not treating for supine hypotension

Slide No.	Lecture Content	Notes

7-27

Abdominal Trauma and Trauma in the Pregnant Patient Summary

The cornerstone of assessing and managing the pregnant and non-pregnant abdominal trauma patient is maintaining a high index of suspicion.

Head Trauma

CHAPTER OBJECTIVES

At the completion of this course the student will be able to:

- Identify the general anatomy of the head.

- Define the physiology and pathophysiology of hypoperfusion, concussion, contusion, laceration, hematoma, and fractures pertinent to the head.

- Define increased intracranial pressure and list the progression of events as pressure rises.

- Define Cushing's triad (response).

- Explain the indications for hyperventilation in the head injury patient.

- Identify the need for cervical spine immobilization with a significant head injury.

- Identify the need for rapid transport of a patient with a decreased level of consciousness from a significant head injury.

Slide No.	Lecture Content	Notes

8-1 A   *Title Slides*

8-1 B

8-2   *Lesson 8 Objectives*

8-3   FOCUS: **Review objectives**

- Discuss the anatomy of the head and brain.
- Discuss the pathophysiology of head trauma.
- Discuss the assessment and treatment of a patient with a suspected head injury.
- Identify the following conditions:
  - Cerebral concussion   – Epidural hematoma
  - Cerebral contusion   – Subdural hematoma
  - Skull fracture   – Intracerebral bleeds

8-4   *Head Injuries*

8-5   FOCUS: **Discuss statistics of head injuries**

- Head injuries are the leading cause of trauma deaths.
- Victims of head injuries are commonly young adults.
- Head injuries are further complicated by drug and alcohol abuse.
- Head injuries are common in multisystem trauma patients.
- Missed or improperly treated head injuries often result in death.
- Use of alcohol and/or drugs complicates assessment.

8-6   *Anatomy and Physiology*

FOCUS: **Identify and discuss the anatomy and physiology of the head and brain**

- Pia mater, arachnoid membrane, dura mater, and skull

8-7   *Potential Spaces*

8-8   FOCUS: **Discuss the potential spaces located within the skull**

- The skull contains a variety of potential spaces.
- They are located between the layers surrounding the brain.
  - Epidural space
  - Subdural space
  - Subarachnoid space

What is normally located within these spaces?

8-9   *Brain Anatomy*

FOCUS: **Identify and discuss the major anatomy of the brain**

- Brain stem, cerebellum, cerebrum, and medulla

Slide No.	Lecture Content	Notes

8-10   *Pathophysiology*

8-11   FOCUS: **Discuss the pathophysiology of intracranial pressure (ICP) and cerebral perfusion**

- $PaCO_2$ has a profound effect on cerebral blood flow.
- When $PaCO_2$ rises above normal, cerebral blood vessels dilate, increasing blood flow.
- When $PaCO_2$ decreases dramatically, the cerebral vessels constrict, decreasing blood flow.
- A $PaCO_2$ may temporarily decrease the ICP, but at a cost!
- What is the immediate impact of decreasing the flow of blood to the brain?
- Monitoring of CO_2 is needed to maintain cerebral blood flow.

What effects will increased $PaCO_2$ have during a head injury?

Increased $PaCO_2$ levels cause increased cerebral bleeding. Increased bleeding leads to increased ICP. Increased ICP leads to brain tissue damage and/or herniation.

8-12   *Intracranial Pressure*

FOCUS: **Discuss the pathophysiology of ICP and the effect on brain tissue**

- The skull is a rigid boxlike structure. If pressure increases within the cranial vault there is no room for expansion.
- This raises the ICP.
- As ICP increases, blood flow to the brain decreases.
- Anaerobic metabolism begins to take place.

8-13   *Autoregulation*

FOCUS: **Discuss the pathophysiology of cerebral perfusion and compensatory mechanisms**

- The brain senses a decrease in oxygenation.
- In an attempt to increase its own oxygenation, the brain stimulates the cardiovascular system to increase blood flow by increasing blood pressure.
- The respiratory system also attempts to increase oxygen.
- Finally, the pulse decreases.

If the ICP continues to rise, what eventually happens to the brain?

8-14   *Head Trauma—Level One*

FOCUS: **Discuss the pathophysiology of level one head trauma and the effects on patients**

- Decorticate posturing: flexion of upper extremities; extension of torso and legs
- Pupils mid-sized and reactive
- Cheyne-Stokes breathing

Slide No.	Lecture Content	Notes

8-15 *Head Trauma—Level Two*

FOCUS: **Discuss the pathophysiology of level two head trauma and the effects on patients**

- Decerebrate posturing: extension of upper extremities, torso and legs
- Pupils mid-sized and fixed
- Central neurogenic hyperventilation

8-16 *Head Trauma—Level Three*

FOCUS: **Discuss the pathophysiology of level three head trauma and the effects on patients**

- Flaccid, does not react to pain
- Pupils fixed and dilated
- Ataxic (medullary) breathing
- Or, apnea

8-17 *Head Trauma—Pitfall*

FOCUS: **Review pitfalls**

It is common to see more than one level of head trauma with a single head injury patient.

8-18 *Stages of Increasing ICP*

FOCUS: **Discuss and compare three levels of head trauma patients**

8-19 *Cushing's Triad*

FOCUS: **Discuss components of Cushing's triad**

What do you think happens to the patient's level of consciousness (LOC) as ICP increases?

8-20 *Assessment*

FOCUS: **Components of assessment of a suspected head injured patient**

- Trauma patient assessment
- Identify critical vs. noncritical patients
- Evaluate mechanism of injury
- Level of consciousness
- Glasgow Coma Scale score

8-21 *AVPU*

FOCUS: **Discuss the AVPU method of assessing level of consciousness**

Slide No.	Lecture Content	Notes

8-22 *Glasgow Coma Score*

8-23 FOCUS: **Discuss and apply components of the Glasgow Coma scoring**

Table for Glasgow Coma scoring

8-24 *Scenario*

FOCUS: **Present scenario to participants; identify kinematics, global assessment**

You are called to a motorcycle crash. The police tell you they were chasing the patient at a high rate of speed when he failed to negotiate a corner and crashed. As you approach, you see a large male lying supine on the ground. He is wearing a badly scratched helmet, and his respirations are noisy and rapid.

8-25 *Glasgow Coma Score*

8-26 FOCUS: **Continue with presentation of scenario and allow interaction by participants concerning rapid assessment and life-threatening treatment**

- A—Snoring respirations
- B—Rapid
- C—Rapid, bounding pulse
- D—Responsive to painful stimuli, pupils fixed at 4 mm
- Vitals: Pulse 124, RR 38, BP 86/palpation
- What is this patient's problem?
- How are you going to care for him?
- What are this patient's chances of recovery?

8-27 *Scenario*

FOCUS: **Present scenario to participants; focus on history of injury**

You are asked to see a 14-year-old female patient who was knocked unconscious while playing basketball. She hit her head on the floor while diving for a shot. On your arrival, you find a conscious patient complaining of a headache. The coach tells you, "She was unconscious for about a minute then woke up."

8-28 *Findings*

FOCUS: **Continue with presentation of scenario and allow student interaction**

- A—Open
- B—Normal, good BS
- C—Normal
- D—Alert and oriented × 3, PEARL
- Vitals: Pulse 90, RR 16, BP 114/66

What is this patient's problem? What will you do to treat her?

Slide No.	Lecture Content	Notes

8-29   *Scenario*

FOCUS: **Present scenario to participants; discuss history and assessment**

Your patient is a 24-year-old female who was riding a motorcycle off-road when she lost control and crashed. Her friend tells you she was unconscious, woke up, then became unresponsive again. On your arrival, she is still unresponsive.

Given this presentation what do you think her diagnosis would be?

8-30   *Findings*

FOCUS: **Continue with scenario and allow participant interaction**

- A—Open
- B—Cheyne-Stokes, breath sounds clear
- C—Pulse normal, no external bleeding
- D—Responsive to painful stimuli
- Vitals: Pulse 58, RR 28 and irregular, BP 152/98

How are you going to treat this patient? Where do you suspect her bleeding is taking place?

8-31   *Scenario*

FOCUS: **Present scenario to participants, allow interaction, and emphasize history**

You are responding to the home of an unresponsive female patient whose family states that they could not awaken her this morning. The history reveals that she sustained a blow to the head yesterday while playing softball.

What is her problem? Where is she bleeding?

- Suspect subdural bleeding.

8-32   *Head Trauma Summary*

Rapid assessment and aggressive treatment of the suspected head-injured patient is the cornerstone of management and should be followed with prompt transport to a facility that is capable of treating severe head injuries.

Spinal Trauma

CHAPTER OBJECTIVES

At the completion of this course the student will be able to:

- Describe the incidence, morbidity, and mortality of spinal injuries in the trauma patient.

- List in order of frequency, four major activities producing spinal trauma in adults.

- List in order of frequency, three major activities producing spinal trauma in pediatric patients.

- List at least four specific mechanisms that can cause spinal injuries.

- Predict spinal injuries based on mechanism of injury.

- Define neurologic spinal shock.

- Describe the pathophysiology of neurologic spinal shock.

- Demonstrate a clear understanding that three indications of spinal trauma must be assessed: (1) mechanism of injury, (2) the presence of other injury due to violent force, (3) specific signs of spinal trauma.

- Discuss the assessment findings associated with spinal injuries.

- Differentiate between spinal injuries based on the assessment and clinical criteria.

- List at least four specific signs or symptoms of spinal trauma.

- Demonstrate a clear understanding that spinal trauma may be asymptomatic, occult, and without neurologic deficits.

- Identify the major goal of spinal trauma management.

Slide No.	Lecture Content	Notes

9-1 A   *Title Slides*

9-1 B

9-2   *Lesson 9 Objectives*

FOCUS: **Review objectives**

- Review spinal anatomy and physiology.
- Identify mechanisms that have a high incidence for spinal trauma.
- Identify the findings that are often consistent with spinal trauma.
- Demonstrate a clear understanding of the assessment and management of spinal trauma and neurogenic shock.

9-3   *Introduction*

FOCUS: **Discuss the priorities of recognition and implications for patients with cord damage**

- Spinal trauma must be recognized early.
- Mismanagement can result in paralysis.
- Paralysis can mean complete, lifelong disability.
- Financial impact of cord injury amounts to $1.25 million over a patient's lifetime.

9-4   *Spinal Cord Injuries*

FOCUS: **Discuss incidence and causes of cord injuries**

15,000 to 20,000 spinal cord injuries occur each year. The most common age of injury is 16 to 35 years of age.
   Causes:

- MVCs   48%
- Falls   21%
- Penetrating trauma   15%
- Sports injuries   14%

9-5   *Vertebral Anatomy*

FOCUS: **Describe the anatomy of the vertebrae and the fact that various portions can be injured resulting in boney damage, with or without cord damage**

9-6   *Vertebral Column*

FOCUS: **Describe the breakdown of the vertebral column while emphasizing that damage is likely to occur at each of the curves in the spine ("breaking the s")**

9-7   *Pathophysiology*

FOCUS: **Associating assessment findings to damaged nerve tracts**

Damage to the cord or nerve tracts results in:

- Paralysis
- Paresthesia
- Weakness
- Numbness
- Pain

Slide No.	Lecture Content	Notes

9-8

Assessment

FOCUS: **Associating assessment findings to level of cord involvement**

- Use the dermatome map as a guide to the level of cord involvement.
- Know what additional structures may be involved.

9-9

Other Assessment Findings

FOCUS: **Assessment findings may not be the same on each side of the body, but cord injury could still be the cause**

- Incomplete spinal cord lesions may present with unusual findings
  - For example, lack of motor ability in one leg with lack of pain sensation in the other leg due to damage to tracts on one or both sides of the cord.
- Lack of neurologic deficit—vertebral damage can produce cord injury.

9-10

Causes of Spinal Cord Trauma

FOCUS: **Associate types of cord damage to causes or mechanism**

- MVCs
- Diving injuries
- Sports injuries
- Falls from heights

What type of cord injury is likely in each of the above?

9-11

Scenario

FOCUS: **Correlate up-and-over with frontal impact and windshield damage—C-spine damage possible**

You are called to the scene of an MVC. As you arrive you see that collision was a one car vs. tree frontal impact. The vehicle has minor front-end damage. The windshield is spiderwebbed, and the driver's only complaint is neck pain.

What type of injury pattern do you expect to find in this patient?

9-12

Findings

FOCUS: **Stable patients with positive neurologic findings—adequate time to administer splinting device**

- A—Open, clear
- B—Normal, breath sounds clear
- C—Good, strong radial pulse
- D—Alert and oriented × 3, good motor and sensory function in extremities, complains of neck pain
- E—Abrasion on forehead
- Vitals: Pulse 98, RR 18, BP 122/P

Slide No.	Lecture Content	Notes

9-13   *Management*

FOCUS: **Complete spinal immobilization**

How are you going to treat this patient?

Pitfall: Using rapid extrication for all patients

9-14   *Scenario*

FOCUS: **Mechanism: fall is three times the patient's height and he hit head first, so significant head and spine trauma are possible**

You are called to the scene of a construction site where a worker has fallen from a second story roof. Bystanders tell you that he struck his head first. His chief complaint is neck pain. He is unable to move his extremities.

9-15   *Findings*

FOCUS: **Need to continually reassess as swelling at cord level can cause condition to worsen—need to assist ventilations, may need to intubate**

- A—Open
- B—Respiratory rate slightly increased, breath sounds clear
- C—Radial pulse 100, no bleeding noted
- D—Alert and oriented × 3, unable to move extremities

During your 45-minute transport, the patient starts to complain of increasing respiratory difficulty. This progresses to a severe problem.

9-16   *Management*

FOCUS: **Treatment**

How are you going to treat this patient?

9-17   *Scenario*

FOCUS: **Present scenario; allow students to voice their approach**

You are called to the scene of an incident where a person riding in the back of a pickup truck was ejected when the truck hit a bump in the road. Upon arrival you find a 23-year-old male lying in the road. He appears confused and disoriented. You smell alcohol on his breath.

9-18   *Findings*

FOCUS: **Causes of decreased BP could be hypovolemia or neurogenic shock**

- A—Open, clear
- B—Rapid, breath sounds clear
- C—Weak radial pulse
- D—Responsive to verbal stimuli, unable to move his lower extremities
- Vitals: Pulse 128, RR 28, BP 90/66

Slide No.	Lecture Content	Notes

9-19

Management

FOCUS: **Treatment**

Why is this patient's BP so low? How are you going to care for this patient?

   Encourage discussion. Review management of neurogenic shock and hypovolemia.

9-20

Neurogenic Shock

FOCUS: **Review neurogenic shock**

- Hypotension associated with cervical or high thoracic spinal cord injury
- Loss of vasomotor tone below injury
  - Vasodilation of extremities and viscera
  - Skin warm and dry below injury
- Loss of sympathetic tone to heart
  - Bradycardia

Pitfall: Rule out hypovolemia as the cause of the hypotension.

9-21

Scenario

FOCUS: **Present scenario; allow students to voice their approach**

You are called to the scene of a collision in which a semi apparently struck a car, broadside. You note major damage to the passenger side of the car, and its driver is your only patient. The driver is unresponsive and the scene is safe.

9-22

Findings

FOCUS: **Present and assess findings; discuss how to proceed.**

- A—Open
- B—Rapid, shallow; breath sounds clear
- C—Radial pulse absent, rapid carotid, no external bleeding
- D—Responsive to painful stimuli only
- E—Skin cool, pale, diaphoretic

9-23

Management

FOCUS: **Management of a critical trauma patient with potential for spine involvement**

- How are you going to manage this patient?
- Is this patient a candidate for rapid extrication?
- What are the limitations of rapid extrication?

Pitfall: Too long on scene extricating critical patients

Review management of critical trauma patients. Allow discussion. Review indications and limitations of rapid extrication.

Slide No.	Lecture Content	Notes

9-24

Scenario

FOCUS: **Present scenario; allow students to voice their approach**

You are called to the scene of a collision between a car and a bicycle. The cyclist is your only patient. He is not wearing a helmet, but he is walking around at the scene. You note severe damage to the bicycle.

9-25

Findings

FOCUS: **Need for standing immobilization**

- A—Open
- B—Shallow and a little fast; BS clear
- C—Radial pulse strong and slightly rapid; no major bleeding noted
- D—Alert and oriented × 3, no neurologic deficits, complains of pain all over
- E—Significant "road rash" to left side of body, obvious fractured left clavicle

9-26

Management

FOCUS: **Treatment**

How are you going to treat this patient?

Pitfall: Not immobilizing an ambulatory patient.

9-27

Scenario

FOCUS: **Present scenario; allow students to voice their approach**

You are called to the scene of a collision between a motorcycle and a guardrail. The motorcyclist is your only patient. Bystanders report a frontal impact at high speed. The driver is on the ground about 20 feet from the point of impact and is wearing a badly damaged helmet. The scene is safe.

9-28

Findings

FOCUS: **Present and assess findings; discuss how to proceed**

- A—Noisy, gurgling
- B—Rapid, shallow, BS noisy due to upper airway problems
- C—Radial pulse absent, fast carotid, no external bleeding
- D—Responds to painful stimuli only
- E—Angulated left forearm injury. Deformity of left thigh.

9-29

Management

FOCUS: **Discuss management**

How are you going to manage this patient?

Discuss helmet indications.

9-30

Spinal Summary

Patient findings may be varied or negative, so let patient needs dictate the immobilization technique until spinal cord injury can be ruled out.

Musculoskeletal Trauma

CHAPTER OBJECTIVES

At the completion of this course the student will be able to:

- List the four groups used to classify patients with extremity injuries and relate this to priority of care.

- Describe the primary and secondary surveys as related to extremity trauma.

- List the five major pathophysiologic problems that require management in extremity injuries.

- Indicate an understanding of the relationship between hemorrhage and open and closed fractures.

- List the four primary signs and symptoms of extremity trauma; list other signs and symptoms that can indicate less obvious extremity injury.

- Explain the management of extremity trauma, especially in the presence of life-threatening injuries.

- Indicate an understanding of splints and splinting methods.

- Describe the special considerations involved in femur fracture management.

- Describe the management of amputations.

Slide No.	Lecture Content	Notes

10-1 A
10-1 B
Title Slides

10-2
Lesson 10 Objectives
FOCUS: **Review objectives**
- Review musculoskeletal anatomy and physiology.
- Discuss the pathophysiology of musculoskeletal trauma.
- Discuss the management of musculoskeletal trauma in:
  - Isolated trauma
  - Multisystem trauma

10-3
Musculoskeletal Trauma
FOCUS: **Discuss the difference in approach between isolated injury and multisystem trauma**
- The management of musculoskeletal trauma can take different avenues depending on the situation.
- In a simple isolated injury, treatment is aimed at care of the particular appendage.
- In the multisystem trauma patient, management is aimed at treating the life-threatening problems and providing supportive care for the simple musculoskeletal injury.

10-4
Anatomy
FOCUS: **Discuss potential fractures**

Any and all bones in the skeleton are susceptible to injury in trauma.

10-5
Scenario
FOCUS: **Present the scenario and encourage discussion**

Your patient has attempted suicide by cutting his wrist. The police are on the scene and it is safe. On your arrival you observe an awake and oriented male patient. Your primary survey findings show no life-threatening problems. On secondary survey you find a longitudinal incision over the radial artery. Bleeding is moderate.

10-6
Discussion
FOCUS: **In this case the life threat is not great**
- What type of injury does this patient have?
- What ways are there to control the bleeding?
- Does this injury require rapid packaging and transport?
- What other types of injuries to the skin are there?
- Can these types of injuries be life threatening?

The greater threat is that the wound is self-inflicted. Often the musculoskeletal trauma will draw our attention to a more serious problem.

Slide No.	Lecture Content	Notes

10-7

Scenario

FOCUS: **Present scenario and encourage discussion**

You are called to a football game for a patient who was hit in his thigh by the helmet of another player. You find an alert, oriented patient who is complaining of right upper leg pain. Primary survey reveals no life-threatening conditions. On secondary survey you find an angulation of the affected thigh, with swelling in the area.

10-8

Discussion

FOCUS: **Encourage discussion with emphasis on how injuries like this, although musculoskeletal, are life threats**

- What type of injury does this patient have?
- How much blood can this patient lose from this injury?
- Could this injury alone cause enough blood loss to cause shock?
- How would you manage this injury?

10-9

Scenario

FOCUS: **Present the scenario and encourage discussion**

You respond to a patient who has been pinned between a pickup truck and a loading dock. On your arrival the truck has been moved and your patient is lying on the ground. He is complaining of pain in his pelvis. Your primary survey shows early signs and symptoms of shock. When you gently stress his pelvis, crepitis is noted and he screams in pain.

10-10

Discussion

FOCUS: **The emphasis again is on a life-threatening musculoskeletal problem**

- What is this patient's problem?
- Is this patient in need of rapid treatment and transportation?
- How are you going to treat him?

In this case, the pelvic fracture has a great potential for serious internal bleeding. Encourage discussion on appropriate treatment.

10-11

Scenario

FOCUS: **Present the scenario and encourage discussion**

You respond to a pedestrian who has been struck by a car. On arrival you find a 63-year-old woman unresponsive on the pavement. As you get closer, you see obvious angulation deformities of her legs, including an open fracture.

10-12

Findings

FOCUS: **Discuss findings with students**

- A—Open, clear
- B—Rapid, lung sounds clear

Slide No.	Lecture Content	Notes

- C—Pulse rapid, weak; moderate hemorrhage from leg
- D—Responsive to pain
- Vitals: Pulse 132, RR 30, BP 88/P

10-13

Discussion

FOCUS: **Discuss treatment with students**

- What are your priorities of care?
- How are you going to treat this patient?
- Is rapid transport indicated?

Emphasize that although the injury is dramatic in appearance, the life threat may be minimal.

10-14

Summary

- Do not splint simple musculoskeletal trauma before evaluating patients for life-threatening injuries.
- To do so would result in well-splinted cadavers arriving at emergency departments.
- In the multi-system trauma patient, most musculoskeletal trauma can be splinted with a long backboard.

10-15

Musculoskeletal Summary

Assess and treat all life-threatening trauma before isolated musculoskeletal trauma!

Thermal Trauma: Injuries Produced by Heat and Cold

CHAPTER OBJECTIVES

At the completion of this course the student will be able to:

- List basic criteria for assessing burn severity.

- List two life-threatening injuries resulting from burns that require prehospital treatment.

- List five signs that indicate inhalation injury and possible respiratory sequelae after a burn injury.

- Define the rule of nines for adult and pediatric patients.

- List key assessment and management elements for chemical and electrical burns.

- Identify and differentiate between critical and noncritical hyperthermia.

- List the major elements of management of hyperthermia from different causes.

- Define superficial and deep frostbite and explain the management of each.

- Identify and detail the management of patients in primary and secondary hypothermia.

- Explain the difference between immersion and submersion hypothermia and the management of each.

Slide No.	Lecture Content	Notes

11-1 A
11-1 B

Title Slides

11-2

Lesson 11 Objectives

FOCUS: **Review objectives**

- Identify, manage, and differentiate critical and noncritical burns.
- Identify the priorities for managing chemical burns.
- Discuss assessment and care of carbon monoxide inhalation.
- Address the priorities for assessing and managing heat-related illness.
- Discuss the priorities for assessing and managing hypothermia.

11-3

Anatomy and Physiology

FOCUS: **Discuss anatomy and physiology of soft tissue**

- Epidermis
  - Outermost layer
- Dermis
  - Nerve endings, blood vessels
- Subcutaneous
  - Elastic and fibrous tissues, fatty deposits

11-4

Illustration of Burn Depths

FOCUS: **Review burn depth and tissue involvement with visual chart**

- Superficial (first degree)
- Partial thickness (second degree)
- Full thickness (third degree)

11-5

Rule of Nines Illustration

FOCUS: **Discuss the importance of total body surface area (TBSA) and the difference between children and adults**

Why does the Rule of Nines change for children?
   Different proportional body surface areas (i.e., larger head).

11-6

Scenario

FOCUS: **Allow participants to respond to the scenario and questions posed**

You are called to care for a patient who has been burned while fueling his lawn mower. As you approach you see a 32-year-old male with a smoldering right arm. He appears to be in intense pain.
   What are you going to do first?

Slide No.	Lecture Content	Notes

11-7

Findings

FOCUS: **Allow participants to respond to the information provided on slide in regard to scenario**

- A—Clear
- B—Normal, clear BS
- C—Normal pulse, no external bleeding
- D—Alert, oriented × 3
- E—Bright red skin with blisters on entire upper and lower right arm
- Vitals: Normal

11-8

Discussion

FOCUS: **Discuss findings**

What thickness is this burn?

- Superficial (first degree) and partial thickness (second degree) due to blisters and pain—dermis involved

What percent body surface area (BSA) is burned?

- 9% BSA involved

How are you going to treat this patient?

- Assure safety, stop the burning, apply moist dressings
- Why do second degree burns hurt the most?
  - Partial thickness burns are more painful due to nerve ending involvement.

11-9

Treatment

11-10

FOCUS: **Describe burn depth and treatment considerations**

- The first priority is to stop the burning.
- Superficial (first degree)
  - Generally no field treatment needed
- Partial thickness (second degree)
  - Burns of less than 10% can be treated with moist dressings. If over 10% of the body is burned, wet dressings should be avoided due to hypothermia risk. IV analgesics for pain relief may be used if indicated.
- Full thickness (third degree)
  - Dry dressings
- Fluid therapy as indicated

11-11

Scenario

FOCUS: **Allow participants to interact with scenario**

You respond to a structure fire. On your arrival you see a victim who has just been removed from the house and appears unresponsive.

What are your first priorities?

- Airway management is first priority as always.

Slide No.	Lecture Content	Notes

11-12 *Findings*

FOCUS: **Continue to encourage student interaction with the scenario**

- A—Stridor noted, oral mucosa appears red
- B—Rapid, breath sounds—rhonchi in all fields
- C—Weak rapid pulse, no external bleeding noted
- D—Unresponsive
- E—Partial thickness burns of upper chest (9% BSA)

What problems does this patient have? How does carbon monoxide poisoning present?

11-13 *Possible Injuries*

FOCUS: **Allow continued interaction with this scenario**

- Burns
- Upper airway swelling secondary to inhalation of superheated gases
- Carbon monoxide (CO) poisoning
- Trauma related to falls or building collapse

Why is he showing signs and symptoms of shock?

- Signs and symptoms of shock are secondary to the received trauma, not the burns. Burns, alone, rarely cause shock in the prehospital arena.

How are you going to treat him?

- Aggressive airway management to include high flow oxygen
- Treatment of underlying blunt trauma
- Fluid therapy as indicated

11-14 *Special Burn Situations*

FOCUS: **Discuss the special problems associated with chemical burns**

Chemical burns:

What is different about these burns?

- Contact agent will continue to burn until removed.

How would you treat chemical burns?

- Removal of agent from contact is primary goal.
- Removal may be accomplished by brushing away dry chemicals and flushing all other agents with copious amounts of water.
- Transport patient to an appropriate care facility. Inappropriate attempts to neutralize agents can make the burn worse.

11-15 *Electrical Burns*

FOCUS: **Discuss pathophysiology of electrical burns and treatment**

- Direct contact
- Arc injuries
- Flash burns

Slide No.	Lecture Content	Notes

How do you manage these injuries?

Injuries:

- Direct contact—grasping electrical source
- Arc injuries—electrical energy exiting the body, going to ground
- Flash burns—secondary "halo" burn caused by electrical energy exiting the body

Treatment:

- Safely remove patient from the source.
- Stop the burning if necessary.
- Cutaneous burns are treated the same as any thermal burn.
- Many electrical injuries will not be visible.
- What you see is not what you get!!

11-16 Patients Requiring Burn Centers

FOCUS: **Discuss situations that may require treatment at a burn center**

- Burns complicated by respiratory tract injuries
- Partial thickness burns of 30% BSA or greater
- Full thickness burns of 10% BSA or greater
- The young and elderly patients
- Preexisting medical conditions
- Burns of specialty areas

Specialty areas may include:

- Face
- Hands
- Feet
- Genitalia
- Major flexion areas

Discuss local protocol for burns if needed.

11-17 General Treatment

FOCUS: **Discuss general treatment outline for thermal injuries**

- Do not become a victim yourself.
- Airway management and oxygenation are critical.
- Early shock after burns points to other injuries.
- Avoid hypothermia.
- Provide fluid therapy as indicated by the BSA involved (Parkland formula).
- Transport the patient to an appropriate facility.

11-18 Subtitle Slide

Environment injuries

Slide No.	Lecture Content	Notes

11-19 *Scenario*

FOCUS: **Present scenario and allow participants to interact with comments and questions**

You respond to a construction site for a male with an unspecified illness. It is a 90° F day with 90% humidity. Your patient has been working in an enclosed area. Workers report that they found the patient collapsed and confused.

- What are you going to do now?

11-20 *Discussion*

FOCUS: **Discuss scenario**

- What are your concerns?
- What places this patient at high risk for a heat emergency?
- How would you treat him?

11-21 *Other Heat Injuries*

FOCUS: **Discuss signs and symptoms of heat-related injuries**

List the signs, symptoms and likely involvement of each of the following:

- Heat cramps
- Heat exhaustion
- Heat stroke

11-22 *Hypothermia*

FOCUS: **Discuss effects of hypothermia on body systems**

Hypothermia begins when the body temperature reaches 95° F (35° C):

- Shivering begins
- Heart rate, respirations, and BP begin to decrease

Below 90° F (32° C):

- CNS impairment

Below 82° F (28° C):

- Ventricular fibrillation

11-23 *Scenario*

FOCUS: **Present scenario and allow participant interaction**

You respond to the scene where a 34-year-old male has fallen into a sewer. You are on-scene, when after 10 minutes, the rescue team brings up a limp body.

Slide No.	Lecture Content	Notes

11-24

Findings

FOCUS: **Continue interaction from scenario**

- A—Water in airway
- B—Not breathing
- C—Very slow, weak carotid pulse
- D—Unresponsive
- E—Wet clothes removed
- Vitals: Pulse 28, RR 0, BP unobtainable

How are you going to resuscitate this patient?

- Prolonged resuscitation efforts are indicated.
- Avoid rough handling of the patient.
- Pharmacologic therapy may be ineffective until core temperature is near normal.

11-25

Pitfalls

FOCUS: **Discuss potential mishandling/treatment of hypothermic patients**

- Rough handling
- External warming vs. core rewarming
- They are not dead until they are warm and dead!

11-26

Thermal Trauma Summary

The key to caring for thermal injuries is observing safety, protecting damaged tissue, and preserving normal body temperature without ignoring other life-threatening conditions.

Considerations in Pediatric and Geriatric Trauma

CHAPTER OBJECTIVES

At the completion of this course the student will be able to:

- Identify the unique differences in injury patterns for children.

- Demonstrate an understanding of the special importance of managing the airway and restoring adequate tissue oygenation in pediatric patients.

- Identify the quantitative vital signs for children.

- Demonstrate an understanding of management techniques for the variety of injuries found in pediatric patients.

- Calculate the Pediatric Trauma Score.

- Identify the signs of pediatric trauma suggestive of child abuse.

- Demonstrate an understanding of the differences in the mechanism of injury for the elderly.

- Identify the variables in the pathophysiology of aging.

- Demonstrate an understanding of the special considerations in assessing the elderly.

- Understand the importance of identifying any preexisting medical conditions.

- Demonstrate an understanding of the effects of medications taken by the elderly.

- Communicate appropriately with the elderly.

- Define implied consent and explain the usually limited role of third-party powers in trauma scene decision making.

- Identify the signs and symptoms of abuse and neglect in the elderly.

Slide No.	Lecture Content	Notes

12-1 A   *Title Slides*

12-1 B

12-2   *Lesson 12 Objectives*

FOCUS: **Review objectives**

- Identify injury patterns unique to geriatric and pediatric patients.
- Identify anatomical differences in pediatric patients and changes in geriatric patients.
- Discuss the importance of history in pediatric and particularly geriatric patients.
- Discuss management techniques for pediatric and geriatric patients.

12-3   *Life Span Development*

FOCUS: **Discuss body system changes that occur with age**

- Our bodies and body systems grow and develop throughout our lifetime.
- In the young, body systems develop and mature.
- In the elderly, body systems begin to show the effects of aging.

12-4   *Concerns in Common*

FOCUS: **Highlight concerns in the airway system and with shock in the elderly and young patient**

- The anatomical differences in the pediatric airway and respiratory complications in geriatric patients
- Poor compensation and overall response to shock in both the elderly and young

12-5   *Subtitle Slide*

Trauma in children

12-6   *Scenario*

FOCUS: **Read and discuss scenario**

You respond to a call for an injured child. You arrive to find a 5-year-old boy on the ground next to his bicycle.

   What are your concerns for this patient and where would you begin?

12-7   *Assessment*

FOCUS: **Allow participants to discuss the scenario**

- What is the mechanism?
- What injuries do you expect?
- ABCs

Slide No.	Lecture Content	Notes

12-8

Findings

FOCUS: **Discuss findings**

- A—Snoring respirations
- B—Rapid, shallow respirations
- C—Weak, rapid pulse, no obvious bleeding
- D—Responds to painful stimulus
- E—No obvious external trauma

Note: It is 50° F and damp. Does this affect your assessment or treatment?

12-9

Pediatric Trauma

FOCUS: **Discuss pediatric trauma**

- Injury is the most frequent cause of death.
- In pediatric patients 20 to 40% of trauma deaths may be preventable.
- Blunt mechanisms are more common, but instances of penetrating trauma have increased to nearly 15% of injuries.

12-10

Mechanisms in Children

FOCUS: **Review the most common mechanisms of injury for the pediatric population**

- Falls—39%
- Vehicular—38%

12-11

Kinematics in Children

FOCUS: **Discuss the kinematics of pediatric trauma**

- A smaller body absorbs energy in a more concentrated area.
- Softer skeleton

12-12

Airway and Breathing in Children

FOCUS: **Review how pediatric anatomy differs from the anatomy of an adult**

- Smaller airways
- Larger head and tongue
- Potential for immature respiratory muscles, allowing for respiratory fatigue

12-13

Circulation in Children

FOCUS: **Discuss the special nature of pediatric circulation**

- Difficult to determine early signs of shock
- Compensate poorly
- Can deteriorate quickly

Slide No.	Lecture Content	Notes

12-14

Disability in Children

FOCUS: **Difficulty in assessing with younger children**

- May be difficult to fully assess level of consciousness
- Patient's activity level and response to his or her environment may be the best indicators
- Be patient and reassuring

12-15

Hypothermia in Children

FOCUS: **Rapid onset of hypothermia**

- Larger surface area relative to overall body weight and size
- Rapid loss of heat

12-16

Subtitle Slide

Trauma in the elderly

12-17

Geriatric Trauma

FOCUS: **Discuss geriatric population growth and the leading causes of trauma in this population**

- Growing part of the population
- Falls are the leading cause of trauma deaths with motor vehicle crashes second.

12-18

Scenario

FOCUS: **Read and discuss scenario**

You're on the scene with a 70-year-old woman who slipped and fell on an icy stairway at a local church.

- What do you need to know?
- What do you do?

12-19

Findings

FOCUS: **Discuss findings**

- A—Open
- B—Rapid with slight wheeze
- C—Pulse 78 and regular, no obvious bleeding
- D—Lethargic; unable to move legs due to pain
- E—No obvious external trauma

12-20

Airway and Breathing in the Elderly

FOCUS: **Review changes in airway and breathing that come with increased age**

- Respiratory function declines.
- Chest wall is less flexible.
- Alveoli become smaller.
- Lessened ability to clear foreign matter from lungs limits absorption of oxygen.
- Lessened elasticity of lung causes decreased ability to exhale, resulting in CO_2 retention.

Slide No.	Lecture Content	Notes

12-21

Circulation in the Elderly

FOCUS: **Discuss the special nature of geriatric circulation**

- Decreased elasticity plus the thickening and narrowing of blood vessels limit ability to adapt to changes in blood flow.
- This causes poor compensation in response to shock.
- Condition can deteriorate quickly.

12-22

Disability in the Elderly

FOCUS: **Review disabilities common to the elderly**

- Effects of age may present problems in assessing level of consciousness.
- Alzheimer's disease
- Organic brain syndrome
- Sensory changes—vision, hearing, etc.

12-23

Pitfalls with the Elderly

FOCUS: **Discuss pitfalls**

- The possibility of preexisting disease increases with age.
- Medications are a major concern.
- Age and general physical condition greatly influence the body's response to injury.
- When immobilizing, additional padding will be required.

12-24

Managing Pediatrics and Geriatrics

FOCUS: **Discuss management of pediatric and geriatric patients**

- Treat these patients with the same priority considerations: A, B, C, D, E . . .
- When making assessments, consider the patient's age as a complicating factor.
- Potential for rapid deterioration mandates frequent reassessment.

12-25

Children and Elderly Summary

Identify the potential for age-specific complications, while keeping in mind that treatment priorities do not change. Follow patient assessment with continual reassessment.

LESSON 13

Principles in the Care of the Trauma Patient

Slide No.	Lecture Content	Notes
13-1 A	*Title Slides*	
13-1 B	FOCUS: **Putting it all together. This lecture integrates all the concepts previously presented in the course. It is intended to provide a scenario-driven discussion of the total patient care concept.**	
13-2	*Scenario*	
	FOCUS: **Preplanning and communications**	
	The 9-1-1 dispatcher receives a call for a two-car MVC. He determines that there are three patients involved; one is still in the car and is unresponsive. The dispatcher simultaneously dispatches police, fire, and EMS. Moments later the first police unit arrives on the scene and confirms that there are three patients.	
	In your system, what would you do now?	
13-3	*Scenario*	
	FOCUS: **Incident Command System (ICS) and personnel management**	
	You pull into the scene right behind the first engine company. The fire department sets up protection. You, the police sergeant, and the fire captain set up the Incident Command System (ICS). Your partner initiates triage. You request two more EMS units, and your partner informs you that there are two stable patients and one critical patient.	
	How would you manage the manpower that you have on the scene now?	

Slide No.	Lecture Content	Notes

13-4

Scenario

FOCUS: **Need for rapid intervention for life-threatening injuries and need for rapid extrication**

The fire captain assigns two firefighters to treat the patients with minor injuries. Your second unit arrives on the scene and, with your partner, they assess the critical patient. Your partner's primary survey reveals fast, shallow respirations, absent breath sounds on the right, and rapid weak pulse.

What are you going to do now?

13-5

Scenario

FOCUS: **Discuss the particular circumstances of the local class participants; what would they do in this instance, i.e., helicopter, local ED, etc.**

The team that is caring for the critical patient has rapidly extricated her from the car. Her airway is secured, she is hyperoxygenated, and her chest is being decompressed. You have alerted the trauma center to expect a critical patient and that a detailed report will follow. The unit leaves the scene after a total scene time of 9 minutes.

- Would this scenario differ in your system?

13-6

Scenario

FOCUS: **Continuing care and good prehospital care can make a dramatic impact on patient outcome**

The unit arrives at the ED, the patient is transferred, and a report is given to the trauma team. The patient is evaluated and a decision is made to bring her to the operating room for surgery. After 2 weeks in the surgical ICU, and despite complications associated with ARDS, the patient is eventually discharged.

- How do trauma centers and systems save lives?
- What are the advantages of taking this patient to a trauma center?

13-7

Principles Summary

FOCUS: **Putting it all together**

Care of the critically injured trauma patient begins with global evaluation and includes the kinematics of the injury. The cornerstone of prehospital care of the critical patient includes a rapid primary survey to detect life-threatening injuries and aggressive management of those injuries. If indicated, extricate rapidly and transport to an appropriate facility.

Slide No.	Lecture Content	Notes

13-8

Principles Summary

FOCUS: **No one person's job is more, or less, important than any other in the care of the trauma patient. From first responder through specialty physician, everyone must do his or her jobs well to achieve the best possible outcome for the trauma victim.**

- Everybody has an important job to do when it comes to the survival potential of the trauma patient.
- Whether you have 10 years of medical training or 40 hours of EMS training, everyone must do their job for the patient's greatest chance of survival.

13-9

Summary

FOCUS: **Remember that the patient is the most important person in trauma**

- Do your job well—so the patient may have the greatest chance of survival.

SECTION II

Scenarios and Teaching Stations

BASELINE DETERMINATIONS

The scenarios within this section are for use during the baseline stations and the teaching stations while conducting a PHTLS provider program.

OBJECTIVES AND PURPOSE

- Upon completion of this station, the participants, as a group, will have demonstrated their entrance level ability to assess and manage a multisystem trauma patient.
- Upon completion of this station the evaluator will have identified by observation and documentation the group's strengths and weaknesses in the assessment and management of a multisystem trauma patient.

This station is designed to establish a "baseline" of the participant's current ability to manage a multisystem trauma patient. A predetermined baseline scenario is used to allow the participants, as a small group, to perform a "hands on" assessment and initiate a treatment sequence based on previous training. **No other scenario may be substituted for this station.**

This practical exercise should be used to evaluate the group's ability to rapidly assess the trauma patient, render timely and meaningful treatment, and recognize the need for rapid transport. As the group identifies any imminent life threats, they should realize the need to offer immediate treatment prior to following the more conventional rationale of completing a detailed assessment and rendering care based on a thorough series of itemized treatment modes. Documentation of the group's performance can be tracked by using the *Baseline Skill Evaluation Sheet* (found in Section V). The instructional staff should use the findings of this station to help identify the participant's strengths and areas of needed improvement, so that emphasis can be placed on those areas during the course.

EVALUATOR INSTRUCTIONS

As the evaluator, you should read and thoroughly review the Baseline Scenario Scene Summary prior to the course. It is also your responsibility to ensure that the patient is properly prepared for his or her role. Read the *Patient Instructions* included in this section to the patient and be sure he or she understands all instructions. You should brief the patient before the beginning of the baseline station and apart from your participant group.

To begin the baseline scenario, read aloud the *Participant Instructions* included in this section to each group of participants. Next, read the *Baseline Scenario* to each group and allow a brief period for any questions pertinent to the scenario setup. Allow the group as a whole to assess and treat the patient. During this time, the participants' activities should not be interrupted by the evaluator(s), nor should corrective recommendations be made. Once participants have completed the station, and based on their findings and treatment, recite the information from the *Development of the Baseline Scenario Scene* section. If the group is still assessing and/or treating the patient after 10 minutes, stop the scenario. **This station is not designed to be a teaching station,** but rather an opportunity for a self-evaluation by the group members throughout the course of the program.

At the end of the baseline scenario the evaluator should thank the participants for their performance and excuse them from the station. Remember: **NO EVALUATION OR CRITIQUE IS GIVEN AT THIS TIME.** After the participants exit, the evaluator should ready the station for the next group.

PATIENT INSTRUCTIONS

[To be read to the patient by the evaluator]

You are the patient at a trauma assessment station. During this station please respond only as directed by this scenario. Your response may change during the scenario based on the performance of the group. If this is necessary, the evaluator will give you directions for your next response. You will be moulaged to represent the injuries received by the trauma patient. The process of assessment by the group may involve removing certain clothing items. Please wear clothing that can be destroyed and also wear appropriate undergarments (i.e., swimsuit) to prevent embarrassment to yourself or the participants.

Moulaged Injuries

Face:	Marked diaphoresis
	Bruise on forehead
Skin:	Pale in color
	Lips and nail beds cyanotic
Chest area:	Steering wheel imprint and bruising

Presentation

You are found slumped over the steering wheel of your vehicle with the driver's side window rolled down and all doors unlocked.

Response

Neuro:	Awake, confused, and somewhat agitated
Airway:	Patent
Respirations:	Rapid and shallow
Abdomen:	Rigid
Extremities:	Severe pain in left thigh
Verbal:	Repeatedly states "My stomach hurts"

At the conclusion of the scenario the evaluator may ask for your input on the performance of the group, but the evaluator will make the final decision regarding the evaluation of the scenario.

PARTICIPANT INSTRUCTIONS

[To be read to the group by the evaluator]

Hi, my name is _____. This station is a patient assessment station. I will be dispatching your group as members of an ambulance service to the scene of an emergency. All normal equipment found on an ambulance will be at your disposal. Please take the time to look over all your equipment before beginning. If you do not find equipment you believe you may need, please ask for it. It will not be adequate to just verbalize your treatment, such as *"I would take the patient's blood pressure"* or *"I would apply the PASGs."* You must actually perform the skill. If you want a blood pressure reading, I will give it to you after I see you apply the cuff and pump it up. I will try to stay in a position to observe what you assess and perform. If you are feeling for a pulse rate, I will tell you whether or not it is present and its quality if present. If you palpate a body part, I will give you the findings. You are, as a team, to assess the patient and institute appropriate care based on your findings, which may include transport. Please also interact with medical control as you feel is appropriate. Are there any questions regarding what is expected of you as a team?

If there are no questions, or after answering appropriate questions, allow the group to review their equipment and then read the scenario to them.

BASELINE SCENARIO

[To be read to the group by the evaluator]

Your unit is called to the scene of a single motor vehicle crash. Upon arrival you observe an automobile that has struck a concrete bridge abutment head on. Witnesses state that the car was traveling at a high rate of speed (highway speed) when the right front tire blew out. The driver lost control of the vehicle momentarily as it started a 360° spin to the right. The driver appeared to regain control, straightening out the spin, but moments later veered into the bridge abutment.

As you approach the vehicle you notice the front end has received extensive damage with both the fender and hood areas pushed back approximately 12 to 14 inches. The windshield is intact without "starring." The driver is the lone occupant of the vehicle and is slumped over the bent steering wheel. You are able to observe that there is no invasion of the dashboard by the driver. During your observation you note that the driver was wearing his lap belt correctly, but the shoulder harness is stretched behind the headrest so that it would not have to be worn. All other pertinent patient information should be available through your group assessment. *Are there any questions at this time?*

If there are no questions, or after answering appropriate questions, allow the group to begin their assessment of the scenario.

DEVELOPMENT OF THE BASELINE SCENARIO SCENE

The following information is for the use of the evaluation team only. Patient information should be shared with the participants only after they complete the proper assessment or if they request specific information.

Baseline Station Goal

The patient should be rapidly extricated from the vehicle onto a long backboard maintaining manual cervical immobilization, secured to the board, given high-flow supplemental oxygen as soon as possible, and transport initiated to the closest appropriate medical facility within a 10-minute time period. All noncritical treatment should be completed en route. Consideration of tier with an ALS level unit or air transport, if applicable, should be voiced by the group.

Overview of the Scene

The patient is inside the vehicle on the driver's side with the driver's side window rolled down. All doors to the vehicle are unlocked. The scene is safe and there are bystanders with no medical training available to help if needed.

Patient Findings

Neuro:	Awake, confused, and somewhat agitated
Airway:	Patent
Respirations:	Rapid and shallow
Chest:	Steering wheel imprint and bruising, equal breath sounds bilaterally
Pulse:	Palpable weak, rapid (tachycardia) radial
Skin:	Pale in color with cyanotic lips and nail beds, diaphoretic
Abdomen:	Rigid to palpation
Extremities:	Severe pain in left thigh on palpation

PROPER SCENE MANAGEMENT ——————

Establish scene safety.
Consider a request for ALS level care if the team is basic level care.
Consider request for air transport.
Provide continual manual cervical stabilization until the patient's head is secured to the long backboard.
Consider rigid cervical collar application.
Provide high-flow oxygen as soon as possible.
Rapidly extricate patient onto a long backboard.
Secure patient to the long backboard.
Provide rapid transportation to the closest appropriate medical facility.
Complete all other noncritical treatment en route.
Contact medical control.

Initial Vital Signs

[To be shared with the participants only after they complete the proper assessment or procedure]

Blood pressure:	80/palpated
Pulse rate:	120
Respirations:	32

Patient Changes

Time	If the Proper Treatment Does Occur	If the Proper Treatment Does Not Occur
After 3 minutes:	B/P 84, Pulse 120 Respirations 32 LOC unchanged	B/P 70, Pulse 130 Respirations 36 Agitation increases
After 6 minutes:	B/P 90, Pulse 110 Respirations 28 LOC improved	B/P nonpalpable, Pulse 140 (carotid) Respirations 36 Patient becomes nonresponsive
After 8 minutes:	B/P 94, Pulse 110 Respirations 28 2 large bore IVs can be started en route. LOC continues to improve.	Respiratory and cardiac arrest occurs (do not tell participants until they check vital signs)
At 10 minutes:	Stop the scenario. Patient survives.	Stop the scenario. Patient does not survive.

Critical Errors to Watch for

1. Failure to adequately ensure safety of the scene
2. Failure to adequately immobilize/stabilize the cervical spine
3. Failure to provide high-flow oxygen
4. Failure to check the patient's pulse, respiration, and/or level of consciousness
5. Failure to rapidly extricate the patient from the vehicle
6. Failure to secure the patient to a long backboard
7. Failure to begin transportation to the closest appropriate facility
8. Failure to recognize a potential abdominal injury
9. Failure to recognize a potential femur injury
10. Failure to recognize potential internal hemorrhage
11. Failure to recognize potential shock
12. Failure to complete the patient scenario in a 10-minute limit
13. Performance of noncritical interventions at the scene

AIRWAY MANAGEMENT AND VENTILATION SKILLS STATION

INTRODUCTION

Airway management and breathing are the highest priorities when treating a trauma patient. Lack of quality airway management and ventilation skills by the prehospital care provider can lead to increased patient mortality and morbidity. It is paramount that prehospital care providers master the skills outlined in this section in order to properly and effectively manage trauma patients.

The teaching of skills within this station in no way implies that the provider will be able to perform the skills outside of the classroom arena. All partic-

ipants must understand that skills discussed, viewed, and/or practiced within this teaching station may only be performed in a nonclassroom situation when authorized by their certifying or licensing agency.

Equipment List

Item	Quantity
1. #14 or #12 gauge over-the-needle catheters	10
2. #20 gauge over-the-needle catheters	10
3. 10 cc syringe	2
4. Adult intubation manikin	1
5. BVM with reservoir	1
6. Chest decompression manikin or equivalent	1
7. Curved laryngoscope blade	1
8. Disposable gloves (large, medium, small)	1 box of each size
9. Endotracheal tube stylet	2
10. Endotracheal tubes (#7 and #8)	2 of each
11. Laryngoscope handle	1
12. Manikin lubricant	1
13. Oxygen tank	1
14. Oropharyngeal airway	3 (multiple sized)
15. Oxygen connecting tubing	1
16. Nasopharyngeal airway	3 (multiple sized)
17. Rigid cervical collar	1
18. Scissors	1
19. Sharps container	1
20. Stethoscope	1
21. Straight laryngoscope blade	1
22. Tape roll (1 or 2 inch)	2

EVALUATOR INSTRUCTIONS

Give a demonstration/overview of each procedure listed as follows and answer any questions the participants may have regarding the procedures. After demonstration, allow supervised practice of each procedure with individual help as needed.

Participants should perform skills while observing proper body substance isolation and performing other proper safety/performance techniques. Verbalization of performance by the participants will not be acceptable practice.

Participants need only demonstrate those procedures that are within their scope of practice. Participants may choose to demonstrate procedures that are outside of their scope of practice. Participants with limited scope of practice must understand that any procedure observed, practiced, and/or demonstrated by them within a station does not allow them to perform the procedure in a nonclassroom setting without approval of their certifying or licensing agency.

Refer to the fourth edition of *Prehospital Trauma Life Support* (the PHTLS provider textbook), Chapter 4: Airway Management and Ventilation Skills, to find sequenced steps for each procedure.

AIRWAY AND VENTILATION PROCEDURES

Manual Airway Opening Techniques (Basic and Advanced Providers)

Objectives

At the completion of this skill station, the participants will be able to:

1. Identify indications and contraindications for the use of manual airway opening techniques
2. Demonstrate the manual technique of the trauma jaw thrust to open a trauma patient's airway while maintaining manual stabilization and neutral alignment of the patient's head and neck
3. Demonstrate the manual technique of the trauma chin lift to open a trauma patient's airway while maintaining manual stabilization and neutral alignment of the patient's head and neck

Demonstrated Skills by the Participants:

1. Trauma jaw thrust (single-person technique)
2. Trauma chin lift (two-person technique)

Oropharyngeal Airway (OPA) Techniques (Basic and Advanced Providers)

Objectives

At the completion of this skill station, the participants will be able to:

1. Identify indications and contraindications for the use of an oropharyngeal airway
2. Demonstrate an approved method of manually opening the airway of a trauma patient
3. Demonstrate proper placement of an oropharyngeal airway using the tongue-jaw lift insertion method
4. Demonstrate proper placement of an oropharyngeal airway using the tongue blade insertion method

Demonstrated Skills by the Participants:

1. Oropharyngeal airway insertion using the tongue-jaw lift insertion method
2. Oropharyngeal airway insertion using the tongue blade insertion method

Nasopharyngeal Airway (NPA) (Basic and Advanced Providers)

Objectives

At the completion of this skill station, the participants will be able to:

1. Identify indications and contraindications to the use of a nasopharyngeal airway
2. Demonstrate an approved method of inserting a nasopharyngeal airway

Demonstrated Skills by the Participants:

1. Nasopharyngeal airway insertion

Bag-Valve-Mask (BVM) Ventilation
(Basic and Advanced Providers)

Objectives
At the completion of this skill station, the participants will be able to:
1. Identify indications and contraindications to the use of a bag-valve-mask system
2. Demonstrate a manual technique to open a trauma patient's airway while maintaining manual stabilization and neutral alignment of the patient's head and neck
3. Demonstrate insertion of an oropharyngeal or nasopharyngeal airway
4. Demonstrate proper assembly of a bag-valve-mask system to include use of high-flow supplemental oxygen and reservoir
5. Demonstrate the one-person technique to ventilate a trauma patient using a bag-valve-mask system
6. Demonstrate the two-person technique to ventilate a trauma patient using a bag-valve-mask system
7. Demonstrate the three-person technique to ventilate a trauma patient using a bag-valve-mask system

Demonstrated Skills by the Participants:
1. One-person BVM technique
2. Two-person BVM technique
3. Three-person BVM technique

Esophageal Tracheal Double Lumen Airway (ETDLA)
(Basic Providers)

Objectives
At the completion of this skill station, the participants will be able to:
1. Identify indications and contraindications for the use of an ETDLA
2. Demonstrate proper insertion of an ETDLA while maintaining manual stabilization and neutral alignment of the trauma patient's head and neck
3. Demonstrate ventilation and oxygenation of a trauma patient with an ETDLA in place

Demonstrated Skills by the Participants:
1. Insertion of an ETDLA
2. Ventilation with an ETDLA in place

Endotracheal Intubation (Advanced Providers)

Objectives
At the completion of this skill station, the participants will be able to:
1. Identify indications and contraindications for the use of visualized orotracheal intubation
2. Identify indications and contraindications for the use of blind naso-tracheal intubation
3. Demonstrate the proper technique for visualized orotracheal intubation of a trauma patient while maintaining manual stabilization and neutral alignment of the patient's head and neck using the one-person technique
4. Demonstrate the proper technique for visualized orotracheal intubation of a trauma patient while maintaining manual stabilization and

neutral alignment of the patient's head and neck using the two-person technique
5. Demonstrate the proper technique for blind nasotracheal intubation of a trauma patient while maintaining manual stabilization and neutral alignment of the patient's head and neck.
6. Demonstrate the proper technique of ventilating an intubated trauma patient with a bag-valve-mask system while maintaining manual stabilization and neutral alignment of the patient's head and neck

Demonstrated Skills by the Participants:
1. Visualized orotracheal intubation (one-person technique)
2. Visualized orotracheal intubation (two-person technique)
3. Blind nasotracheal intubation (Note: The patient must have his or her own respiratory efforts before attempting this technique.)
4. Ventilation of an intubated patient while maintaining manual stabilization and neutral alignment of the patient's head and neck

Percutaneous Transtracheal Ventilation (PTV) (Optional Skill for Advanced Providers)
Objectives
At the completion of this skill station, the participants will be able to:
1. Identify indications and contraindications to the use of percutaneous transtracheal ventilation
2. Identify the anatomical landmarks used to perform percutaneous transtracheal ventilation
3. Demonstrate the technique of percutaneous transtracheal ventilation

Emergency Needle Thoracostomy (Advanced Providers)
Objectives
At the completion of this skill station, the participants will be able to:
1. State the indications and contraindications to the use of emergency needle thoracostomy
2. Identify the anatomical landmarks for emergency needle thoracostomy
3. Demonstrate the proper technique for emergency needle thoracostomy

Demonstrated Skills by the Participants:
1. Needle decompression of the chest (Note: The evaluator may wish to have the participants use a smaller gauge catheter-over-needle IV to help preserve the practice equipment. Initially, participants should still select the correct size large bore IV.)

PATIENT ASSESSMENT SKILLS STATION
INTRODUCTION

Assessment of the trauma patient is the most important skill a prehospital provider possesses. A complete, comprehensive, and timely assessment and reassessments of the trauma patient will increase the patient's chances of surviving his or her injuries. This assessment must include as much information as possible. Such information could include mechanism of injury, scene conditions, critical indicators, and so on. Each provider should be comfortable with his or her assessment skills in any given situation. Certain trauma patients may have such life-threatening injuries that you may never complete a total assessment. The focus of your assessment will be to initially identify whether you are treating a critical or noncritical patient. A critical trauma patient may cause you to focus all your attention on maintaining the patient's vital signs allowing no time to complete a detailed assessment. While this type of assessment is acceptable for the critical patient, it is unacceptable for the noncritical patient. A thorough and complete assessment and reassessment must be completed whenever indicated.

The teaching of skills within this station in no way implies that the provider will be able to perform the skills outside of the classroom arena. All participants must understand that skills discussed, viewed, and/or practiced within this teaching station may only be performed in a nonclassroom situation when authorized by their certifying or licensing agency.

Equipment List

Item	Quantity
1. Cervical collars	Multiple sizes
2. Dressing and bandaging material	Multiple
3. Eye protection	Each participant
4. Gloves	Multiple sizes
5. Patient	1
6. Pen light	1
7. Scenarios	2 (minimum)
8. Stethoscope	1

EVALUATOR INSTRUCTIONS

Give a demonstration/overview of each procedure listed as follows and answer any questions the participants may have regarding the procedures. After demonstration, allow supervised practice of each procedure with individual help as needed.

Participants should perform skills observing proper body substance isolation and other proper safety/performance techniques. Verbalization of the performance by the participants will not be acceptable practice.

Participants need only demonstrate those procedures that are within their scope of practice. Participants may choose to demonstrate procedures that are outside of their scope of practice. Participants with limited scope of practice must understand that any procedure observed, practiced, and/or demonstrated by them within this station does not allow them to perform the procedure in a nonclassroom setting without approval of their certifying or licensing agency.

Refer to the fourth edition of the PHTLS provider textbook, Chapter 2: Patient Assessment and Management, to find sequenced steps for each procedure.

PATIENT ASSESSMENT PROCEDURES

Patient Assessment (Basic and Advanced Providers)

Objectives
At the completion of this skill station, the participants will be able to:
1. Demonstrate the proper technique for assessing a trauma patient during a given scenario
2. Identify the proper treatment for any deficiencies identified during assessment of a trauma patient in a given scenario

Demonstrated Skills by the Participants:
1. Assessment of a trauma patient
2. Treatment of identified deficiencies found during assessment of a trauma patient

SCENARIO A

You are dispatched to the scene of a bicycle accident. Upon arrival you find a 12-year-old patient sitting on the grass of a front yard. There is one person attending to the patient, and another person approaches you and states that they were the individuals who called for the ambulance. They had witnessed the girl traveling down the sidewalk on her bicycle at a fast rate of speed. She seemed to lose control of the bicycle while trying to turn into the driveway, and she hit a car parked in the driveway. Approaching the patient you learn that the other person attending the child is the patient's parent. The patient is sitting on the ground softly crying and cradling her left forearm in her lap. The patient tells you she was "just goofing around" when she ran into a parked car. She complains of pain in her left wrist and left lower leg. Both extremities exhibit increased pain each time she tries to move. The patient's parent states that the child was not wearing a helmet and has no previous medical history, is not allergic to anything, and is not taking any medications.

Assessment Format for Scenario A

Participant's Assessment	Findings
Scene survey	Scene is safe.
	As described in scenario
Mechanism of injury	Single bicycle crash into a parked car
Initial assessment (primary)	12-year-old patient
	Conscious and alert, softly crying
	Sitting upright on ground holding her left forearm in her lap
	Breathing is adequate.
	Minor abrasions to the patient's left arm and leg without active bleeding
	Small abrasion to the patient's left forehead without active bleeding
	Strong, rapid radial pulse
Critical versus non-critical patient	Noncritical patient
	Further assessment and treatment indicated

Focused assessment (secondary)	Deformity in patient's left wrist and left ankle
	Increased pain in left extremities with movement
	Vital signs are within normal limits.
	Neurovascular checks are normal.
	No other injuries noted
Treatment	Manual stabilization of the patient's head and neck based on mechanism of injury and assessment findings
	Size and apply cervical collar.
	Splint both injured extremities.
	Secure patient to a long backboard (may include use of a short board).
	Transport to the nearest facility.
Reassessment	All findings are within normal limits.

SCENARIO B

Your service is called to the scene of a construction accident. Upon arrival you are led to a patient lying supine on the ground. The patient is being attended to by a group of co-workers. As you approach, the crowd parts and lets you through. You find a 23-year-old male who fell from a broken ladder. Co-workers state that the patient was carrying a bundle of shingles up the ladder when a rung broke causing him to fall approximately 12 feet to the ground landing on his buttocks and then his back. Co-workers have not attempted to move the patient since his fall. The patient is conscious and alert and complains of not being able to move his legs since the fall.

Assessment Format for Scenario B

Participant's Assessment	Findings
Scene survey	Scene is safe.
	As described in scenario
Mechanism of injury	Fall from ladder approximately 12 feet to the ground landing on buttocks, then back
Initial assessment (primary)	23-year-old male
	Conscious and alert
	Lying supine on ground
	Breathing is normal.
	No external hemorrhage noted
	Strong radial pulse noted
	Skin is pale from the mid-abdomen downward.
Critical versus non-critical patient	Noncritical patient
	Further assessment and treatment indicated
Focused assessment (secondary)	No feeling or movement in lower extremities
	Poor circulation in lower abdomen and lower extremities (skin color and delayed capillary refill)
	Pain and tenderness upon palpation to the back (lumbar/thoracic area)
	All other vital signs within normal limits
	No significant past history
	No current medications
	No known allergies

Participant's Assessment	Findings
Treatment	Manual stabilization of the head and neck
	Size and apply cervical collar.
	Transfer to a long backboard and secure.
	Consider supplemental oxygen.
	Consider IV initiation.
	Transport to the nearest facility capable of handling the patient's injuries.
Reassessment	All findings are within normal limits except for loss of feeling and movement of the lower extremities.

SCENARIO C

Your service is dispatched to the scene of a fight at a local barroom. Upon arrival you find the patient lying on the floor of the barroom with the bartender in attendance. The bartender states that the patient got into a fight with another guy after beating him in a pool game. The other player hit the patient in the head with a pool cue several times until the patient fell to the floor. The other player then proceeded to beat the patient's head on the floor for several minutes. The other player then fled from the barroom. The bartender also states that both of the players had been drinking beer for several hours. You find the patient lying on his back on the barroom floor. The patient is nonresponsive to verbal stimulus.

Assessment Format for Scenario C

Participant's Assessment	Findings
Scene survey	Scene is safe.
	As described in scenario
Mechanism of injury	Blunt trauma to the head
Initial assessment (primary)	Male patient (25–30 years old)
	Nonresponsive to verbal stimulus
	Nonresponsive to painful stimulus
	Irregular, noisy respirations (8–14)
	Minor bleeding from multiple scalp lacerations
	Blood seeping from the patient's right ear opening
	Fixed and dilated left pupil
	Slow, weak radial pulse (40)
Critical versus non-critical patient	Critical patient
Focused assessment (secondary)	Deferred until time and resources allow
Treatment	Manual stabilization of the head and neck
	Size and apply cervical collar.
	Secure airway.
	Rapid survey to detect other injuries (none found)
	Transfer and secure to a long backboard.
	High-flow oxygen
	Consider initiation of IV (en route).
	Consider application of PASG (en route).
	Timely transport to an appropriate level trauma facility capable of treating your patient's head injuries

SCENARIO D

Your service is dispatched to the scene of a drive-by shooting. As you approach the scene you are directed by law enforcement to a teenage male patient lying supine on the ground outside of a multiple family housing unit. Law enforcement tells you that the youth is a member of one of the local gangs. They think a member of a rival gang shot the patient. Other law enforcement officers are securing the area while they search for the gunman. The patient is lying on his right side on the ground conscious and alert with his knees drawn to his chest. The patient states over and over that he has been shot.

Assessment Format for Scenario D

Participant's Assessment	Findings
Scene survey	Scene is safe.
	As described in scenario
Mechanism of injury	Gunshots from a medium velocity weapon fired from approximately 12 feet away
Initial assessment	Teenage male patient
	Conscious and alert
	Lying on his right side with knees drawn to chest
	Patient states over and over that he has been shot
	Rapid, shallow respirations
	Weak, rapid carotid pulse (no radial pulse)
	Skin pale in color, cool and damp to touch
	Hemorrhage from four wounds, two smaller wounds (one anterior right chest, one anterior right abdomen), two larger wounds (one posterior right chest, one posterior right abdomen)
	Decreased breath sounds on right side
Critical versus non-critical patient	Critical patient
Focused assessment (secondary)	Deferred until time and resources allow
Treatment	Rapid survey to detect further injuries (none found)
	High-flow oxygen via non/partial rebreather
	Occlusive dressings over chest wounds
	Transfer to long backboard and secure
	Timely transport to appropriate level trauma facility
	Consider initiation of IV(s) en route.
	Consider modified Trendelenberg position (head lower than abdomen).
Reassessment	Increased difficulty breathing
	Consider development of tension pneumothorax and proper treatment
	All other findings remain the same.

SCENARIO E

Your service is dispatched to the scene of a fall. Upon arrival you are directed by a family member to the basement of a home where the elderly resident has fallen down a flight of stairs. The family member states that they had been trying to contact their father by phone for over a day without success. They came over this afternoon to check on him and found him lying at the bottom of the basement stairs. They state that their father lives here by himself and has a past medical history of several transient ischemic attacks (TIAs). The patient takes a blood thinner everyday along with a diuretic. Family members had been unable to move their father after finding him on the floor but did cover him with a blanket. You find the patient lying on his back on the basement floor conscious and alert. The patient tells you he was carrying a chair downstairs yesterday morning when he lost his balance, slipped, and fell down most of the stairs. When he fell he landed on the back of the chair on the left side of his belly. He has been unable to move due to pain in his left hip area and left abdomen. He apologizes for losing control of his bowel and bladder, but he could not move to get to the bathroom or to the telephone.

Assessment Format for Scenario E

Participant's Assessment	Findings
Scene survey	Scene is safe.
	As described in scenario
Mechanism of injury	Fall down flight of stair
	Landing on chair
Initial assessment (primary)	70-year-old male
	Conscious and alert
	Respirations normal
	Weak, rapid radial pulse
	Skin pale in color, cool and damp to the touch
	External rotation and shortening of the left leg
	Bruising over the left upper abdomen
	Urine and feces covering the inside and back of lower extremities
Critical versus non-critical patient	Critical patient (suspect hip fracture with internal abdominal bleeding)
Focused assessment	Deferred until time and resources allow
Treatment	Manual stabilization of the head and neck
	Size and apply cervical collar.
	Apply high-flow oxygen.
	Manual stabilization of left lower extremity
	Rapid survey to detect other injuries (none noted)
	Transfer and secure to a long backboard.
	Timely transport to the nearest appropriate level trauma facility
	Consider application of the PASGs.
	Consider initiation of IV en route.
Reassessment	No changes

PEDIATRIC ASSESSMENT SKILL STATIONS

PURPOSE

To allow the participants an opportunity to assess and treat pediatric trauma patients in a classroom setting.

GOALS

At the completion of this station, each participant will be able to:
1. Complete a comprehensive assessment of a pediatric trauma patient during a given scenario.
2. Treat injuries associated with a pediatric trauma patient.
3. Use pediatric-style treatment equipment.

EVALUATOR INSTRUCTIONS FOR PEDIATRIC ASSESSMENT STATIONS I AND II

Review and demonstrate the techniques for assessing and treating a pediatric trauma patient with the group as a whole. After answering any questions the participants may have regarding the assessment of a pediatric trauma patient, select one of the supplied scenarios and read aloud to the group. Have one individual assume the leader role and assess the patient from the chosen scenario. As much as time allows, have each participant rotate through the leader role and perform an assessment. As the group assesses the patient, provide them with the information supplied for each scenario. The ideal treatment for each scenario is also supplied. Verbalization of invasive procedures will be acceptable. You may choose to select a new scenario for each new leader. Review each scenario you will use with your patient and their role-playing actions prior to beginning your station.

Equipment List for Pediatric Assessment Scenario A

1. Blankets and towels
2. Blood pressure equipment (pediatric)
3. Body substance protection equipment
4. Cervical collars (pediatric)
5. Long bone splints (pediatric)
6. Medic response box
7. PASG (pediatric)
8. Patient (pediatric)
9. Spinal immobilization equipment (pediatric)
10. Stethoscope
11. Straps
12. Supplemental oxygen equipment
13. Tape
14. Traction splint (pediatric)

Pediatric Assessment Scenario A

[To be read aloud to the group]

Your service is called to the scene of a child who fell from a moving vehicle. Upon arrival, bystanders state that the child was riding in the open back of a pickup truck playing with some other children. When the truck rounded the corner, the child fell out. The car traveling behind the pickup slammed on the brakes to avoid hitting the child. The bystanders are unsure if the car missed the child or not. As you approach the patient, you find the child being attended to by a young teenager (the driver of the truck). He tells you that the patient is his 10-year-old cousin. They had been to a family reunion when he took a group of his cousins for a ride in his truck around the neighborhood. They were just going back to the picnic when she fell out. He is also unsure if the car behind him hit or missed his cousin. You find the patient lying in the traveled portion of the street.

Do you have any questions before beginning?

Injuries for Pediatric Assessment Scenario A

Body Area/Function	Injury/Response
Patient presentation	Lying prone
	Arms to the side of head
	Head turned to the side
Head/face	Abrasions to right side of face
	Fixed and dilated left pupil
Chest/abdomen	No injuries
Extremities	Abrasions to both forearms and hands
Level of consciousness	Non-responsive to verbal or painful stimulus
Respirations	Ataxic 8–14/minute
Breath sounds	Clear and equal
Circulation/blood pressure	Slow weak radial pulse (54)
	BP: 74/palpable
History	Not available

Proper Treatment of Pediatric Assessment Scenario A

1. Complete initial (primary) assessment
2. Identify critical patient (closed head injury)
3. Maintain manual immobilization of head and neck
4. Ventilatory support with high-flow oxygen
5. Logroll patient onto long backboard
6. Proper use of padding
7. Complete spinal immobilization
8. Apply supplemental high-flow oxygen if respirations stabilize
9. Timely transport to an appropriate level care facility
10. Interaction with medical control as indicated

Equipment List for Pediatric Assessment Scenario B

1. Blankets and towels
2. Blood pressure equipment (pediatric)
3. Body substance protection equipment
4. Cervical collars (pediatric)
5. Chest decompression equipment
6. Helmet (pediatric)
7. IV supplies
8. Long bone splints (pediatric)

9. Medic response box
10. PASG (pediatric)
11. Patient (pediatric)
12. Spinal immobilization equipment (pediatric)
13. Stethoscope
14. Straps
15. Supplemental oxygen equipment
16. Tape
17. Traction splint (pediatric)

Pediatric Assessment Scenario B

[To be read aloud to the group]

Your service is dispatched to a local dirt track used for sport recreational vehicles on a clear, sunny afternoon. Upon your arrival, you see a large group of individuals looking down a steep embankment. You observe four people carrying a child up to level ground. Witnesses state that the child was operating a "dune buggy" when it failed to negotiate a curve due to loose gravel, went over the embankment, and rolled several times. You estimate that the embankment goes down about 20 feet. After the child is brought up from the embankment and placed in a supine position on the ground, the uncle states that the child was thrown from the vehicle about half-way down. The patient appears to be about 9 years old, is responsive to verbal stimulus, and is still wearing the helmet. The uncle knows of no past pertinent medical history.

Injuries for Pediatric Assessment Scenario B

Body Area/Function	Injury/Response
Patient presentation	Lying supine with helmet on
Head/face	Pupils equal and reactive
Chest/abdomen	Abrasions and bruising to the chest and abdomen areas
Extremities	Closed fracture to the right femur
	Laceration with active venous bleeding left forearm
	Abrasions to both upper extremities
Level of consciousness	Responsive to verbal stimulus
Respirations	Labored 22–24/minute
Breath sounds	Decreased sounds on the left side
Circulation/blood pressure	Rapid, weak radial pulse (124)
	BP: 74/palpable
	Delayed capillary refill
	Skin pale in color
History	None known

Proper Treatment of Pediatric Assessment Scenario B

1. Complete initial (primary) assessment
2. Identify critical patient (possible internal bleeding)
3. Maintain manual immobilization of head and neck
4. Helmet removal

5. Ventilatory support with high-flow oxygen
6. Logroll patient onto long backboard
7. Proper use of padding
8. Complete spinal immobilization
9. Stabilization of femur fracture (traction splint or PASG)
10. Verbalize decompression of suspected pneumothorax (if within the provider's scope of practice)
11. Apply supplemental high-flow oxygen if respirations stabilize
12. Timely transport to an appropriate level care facility
13. Initiation of IV(s) (if within the provider's scope of practice)
14. Interaction with medical control as indicated

Equipment List for Pediatric Assessment Scenario C

1. Blankets and towels
2. Blood pressure equipment (pediatric)
3. Body substance protection equipment
4. Cervical collars (pediatric)
5. Chest decompression equipment
6. Long bone splints (pediatric)
7. Medic response box
8. PASG (pediatric)
9. Patient (pediatric) (may use a CPR mannequin for this scenario)
10. Spinal immobilization equipment (pediatric)
11. Stethoscope
12. Straps
13. Supplemental oxygen equipment
14. Tape
15. Traction splint (pediatric)

Pediatric Assessment Scenario C

[To be read aloud to the group]

Your service is dispatched to a single family home. Upon arrival your unit is greeted by frantic parents who tell you that while they were sitting on the front lawn with their 2-year-old child, a talkative neighbor distracted them. In the few moments of inattention, their baby crawled over the top of a 10-foot high retaining wall next to their driveway. The child fell approximately 5 feet initially, landing on the roof of their car. As they ran to the child, the child rolled from the car onto the concrete driveway, where the child now lies in a supine position covered with a blanket.

Injuries for Pediatric Assessment Scenario C

Body Area/Function	Injury/Response
Patient presentation	Lying supine on driveway
Head/face	Pupils unequal and nonreactive
Chest/abdomen	No injuries noted
Extremities	Minor abrasions
Level of consciousness	Nonresponsive to verbal or painful stimulus
Respirations	Labored 22–24/minute

Breath sounds	Decreased sounds on the left side
Circulation/blood pressure	Rapid, weak brachial pulse (140)
	BP: 74/palpable
	Delayed capillary refill
	Skin pale in color
History	None known

Proper Treatment of Pediatric Assessment Scenario C

1. Complete initial (primary) assessment
2. Identify critical patient (possible head injury and internal bleeding)
3. Maintain manual immobilization of head and neck
4. Ventilatory support with high-flow oxygen
5. Logroll patient onto long backboard
6. Proper use of padding
7. Complete spinal immobilization
8. Verbalize decompression of suspected pneumothorax (if within the provider's scope of practice)
9. Apply supplemental high-flow oxygen if respirations stabilize
10. Timely transport to an appropriate level care facility
11. May consider application of PASG
12. Initiation of IV(s) (if within the provider's scope of practice)
13. Interaction with medical control as indicated

Equipment List for Pediatric Assessment Scenario D

1. Blankets and towels
2. Blood pressure equipment (pediatric)
3. Body substance protection equipment
4. Cervical collars (pediatric)
5. Long bone splints (pediatric)
6. Medic response box
7. PASG (pediatric)
8. Patient (pediatric)
9. Spinal immobilization equipment (pediatric)
10. Stethoscope
11. Straps
12. Supplemental oxygen equipment
13. Tape
14. Traction splint (pediatric)

Pediatric Assessment Scenario D

[To be read aloud to the group]

Your service is dispatched to a second-floor apartment building. Upon entering the apartment, the babysitter states that the 7-year-old child she was caring for somehow got out onto the fire escape while she was talking on the phone. The child fell down the ladder stairs to the first-floor landing. The fire escape is constructed of slated iron, and you estimate the distance from the second floor to the first floor landing to be approximately 15 feet. After the fall, the babysitter picked up and carried the child back upstairs to the couch, where the child is lying in a supine position crying and complaining of stomach pain.

Injuries for Pediatric Assessment Scenario D

Body Area/Function	Injury/Response
Patient presentation	Lying supine on couch
Head/face	Pupils equal and reactive
Chest/abdomen	Minor abrasions
Extremities	Minor abrasions
Level of consciousness	Responsive to verbal stimulus
Respirations	Soft crying
	18–22/minute
Breath sounds	Clear and equal
Circulation/blood pressure	Rapid, weak radial pulse (140)
	BP: 70/palpable
	Delayed capillary refill
	Skin pale in color
History	None known

Proper Treatment of Pediatric Assessment Scenario D

1. Complete initial (primary) assessment
2. Identify critical patient (internal bleeding)
3. Maintain manual immobilization of head and neck
4. Move patient onto long backboard
5. Proper use of padding
6. Complete spinal immobilization
7. Apply supplemental high-flow oxygen if respirations stabilize
8. Timely transport to an appropriate level care facility
9. May consider application of PASG
10. Initiation of IV(s) (if within the provider's scope of practice)
11. Interaction with medical control as indicated

Equipment List for Pediatric Assessment Scenario E

1. Blankets and towels
2. Blood pressure equipment (pediatric)
3. Body substance protection equipment
4. Cervical collars (pediatric)
5. Dressings and bandages
6. Long bone splints (pediatric)
7. Medic response box
8. PASG (pediatric)
9. Patient (pediatric)
10. Scoop-style stretcher
11. Spinal immobilization equipment (pediatric)
12. Splints (pneumatic)
13. Stethoscope
14. Straps
15. Supplemental oxygen equipment
16. Tape
17. Traction splint (pediatric)

Pediatric Assessment Scenario E

[To be read aloud to the group]

Your service is dispatched to a local elementary school for an injured student. Upon arrival, you are directed to the gymnasium. You find a group of students surrounding another student who is lying on the gym floor being attended to by a teacher. The teacher states that the students were climbing a rope when this student fell about 12 feet to the floor. The patient is 10 years old with no known medical history. You find the patient lying on the floor in a supine position with an open fracture of the left ankle with minimal venous bleeding. The patient is conscious and responds to your questions.

Injuries for Pediatric Assessment Scenario E

Body Area/Function	Injury/Response
Patient presentation	Lying supine on gym floor
Head/face	Pupils equal and reactive
Chest/abdomen	No injuries noted
	Complains of increased pain in lower abdomen upon palpation
	Grating and crepitus noted when pelvis is stressed
Extremities	Open fracture of left ankle
Level of consciousness	Responsive to verbal stimulus
Respirations	18–22/minute
Breath sounds	Clear and equal
Circulation/blood pressure	Rapid, weak radial pulse (140)
	BP: 70/palpable
	Delayed capillary refill
	Skin pale in color
History	None known

Proper Treatment of Pediatric Assessment Scenario E

1. Complete initial (primary) assessment
2. Identify critical patient (internal bleeding, possible fractured pelvis)
3. Maintain manual immobilization of head and neck
4. Move patient onto long backboard (consider use of scoop-style stretcher)
5. Proper use of padding
6. Complete spinal immobilization
7. Splint open fracture of left ankle
8. Apply supplemental high-flow oxygen
9. Timely transport to an appropriate level care facility
10. May consider application of PASG
11. Initiation of IV(s) (if within the provider's scope of practice)
12. Interaction with medical control as indicated

Equipment List for Pediatric Assessment Scenario F

1. Blankets and towels
2. Blood pressure equipment (pediatric)
3. Body substance protection equipment
4. Cervical collars (pediatric)
5. Dressings and bandages
6. Long bone splints (pediatric)
7. Medic response box
8. PASG (pediatric)
9. Patient (pediatric)
10. Scoop-style stretcher

11. Spinal immobilization equipment (pediatric)
12. Splints (pneumatic)
13. Stethoscope
14. Straps
15. Supplemental oxygen equipment
16. Tape
17. Traction splint (pediatric)

Pediatric Assessment Scenario F

[To be read aloud to the group]

Your service is dispatched to a local playground for an injured child. Upon your arrival, you are led to a series of wooden structures that include balance beams and pirate ships in the playground area. Under the dragonhead of one of the ships, you find a 12-year-old patient lying supine on the ground. The patient is conscious and alert and states that they were looking for bad pirates when she lost her balance and fell off the ship, landing on the ground. You estimate that the patient fell approximately 8 feet to the gravel-covered ground.

Injuries for Pediatric Assessment Scenario F

Body Area/Function	Injury/Response
Patient presentation	Lying supine on ground
Head/face	No injuries noted
	Pupils equal and reactive
Chest/abdomen	No injuries noted
Extremities	Closed fracture of right distal forearm
	Unable to move lower extremities
	No sensation in lower extremities
Level of consciousness	Responsive to verbal stimulus
Respirations	18–22/minute
Breath sounds	Clear and equal
Circulation/blood pressure	Rapid radial pulse (140)
	BP: 104/palpable
	Normal capillary refill in hand
	Delayed capillary refill in feet
	Skin normal above the naval area
	Skin pale in color below the naval
History	None known

Proper Treatment of Pediatric Assessment Scenario F

1. Complete initial (primary) assessment
2. Identify critical patient (possible spinal cord injury)
3. Maintain manual immobilization of head and neck
4. Move patient onto long backboard (consider use of scoop-style stretcher)
5. Proper use of padding
6. Complete spinal immobilization
7. Splint fracture of right forearm
8. Apply supplemental high-flow oxygen
9. Timely transport to an appropriate level care facility

10. Initiation of IV(s) (if within the provider's scope of practice)
11. Interaction with medical control as indicated

PEDIATRIC IMMOBILIZATION STATION

PURPOSE

To allow the participants an opportunity to immobilize pediatric trauma patients in a classroom setting.

GOALS

At the completion of this station, each participant will be able to:
1. Complete spinal immobilization of a pediatric trauma patient during a given scenario.
2. Use pediatric-styled spinal immobilization equipment.

Evaluator Instructions for Pediatric Immobilization Station

Review and demonstrate the techniques for assessing and immobilizing a pediatric trauma patient with the group as a whole. After answering any questions the participants may have regarding the assessment and immobilization of a pediatric trauma patient, select one of the supplied scenarios and read aloud to the group. Have one individual assume the leader role and assess the patient from the chosen scenario. As much as time allows, have each participant rotate through the leader role and perform an assessment. As the group assesses the patient, provide them with the information supplied for each scenario. The ideal treatment for each scenario is also supplied. You may choose to select a new scenario for each new leader. Review each scenario you will use with your patient and their role-playing actions prior to beginning your station.

Immobilization Technique—Car-Seat Style Restraint Device

1. Whenever possible, leave the child in the seat-style restraint device Check seat for possible fractures—if no obvious fractures, leave child in the seat for immobilization.
2. Regardless of the position of the seat, apply manual stabilization of the patient's head and neck.
   a. Specific technique for manual stabilization will depend on the size of the patient and the number of rescuers available.
      Two-handed technique—one hand positioned on each side of the patient's head from the front or from above.
      One-handed technique—placed under the patient's chin from above the patient with the back of the head resting against the car seat
3. If indicated, open the patient's airway with trauma jaw thrust. Place the seat in an upright position.
   a. Remove any straps holding the child's car seat to the automobile seat.
   b. Leave straps holding the child to the car-seat restraint device.
4. Measure and apply cervical collar if an appropriate size is available.
   a. Rolled towel may be used. Continue to maintain manual stabilization.

5. Place towels, blankets, etc., between the patient and the restraint device.

May need to place padding behind the patient's shoulders and spine to maintain neutral alignment.

Using tape or straps, secure the patient and padding to the car-seat restraint device.

Manual stabilization may be removed after securing the patient's head to the restraint device.

Move the car seat to the ambulance and secure for transport.

Equipment List for Pediatric Immobilization Station Scenarios A, B, and C

1. Blankets and towels
2. Body substance protection equipment
3. Car-seat style restraint device
4. Cervical collars (pediatric/infant)
5. Patient (infant CPR mannequin)
6. Straps
7. Tape

Pediatric Immobilization Station Scenario A

[To be read aloud to the group]

You are dispatched to the scene of a motor vehicle crash. Upon arrival, you find a car and a minivan involved in a head-on impact at a suburban intersection. Bystanders state that other bystanders took the two drivers of the vehicles to the hospital already. As you are about to depart the scene, you hear what sounds like a child crying. Seeing no other children in the immediate area, you search the van. On the back floor of the van you find an infant in a child's car seat lying on its side. The child appears to be around 10 months old and is softly crying. A quick assessment reveals a laceration to the forehead with minimal venous bleeding. You determine that you need to immobilize the child in the car seat.

Pediatric Immobilization Station Scenario B

[To be read aloud to the group]

Your service is dispatched to the scene of a motor vehicle crash. Upon arrival, you find a single vehicle that has struck a light pole head-on. The driver of the vehicle is sitting in the front seat being attended to by another unit. You find the patient's 14-month-old child in the car-seat restraint device strapped in the front seat, facing forward, and the dash is broken immediately in front of the car seat. You have access to the child and observe that there are no obvious injuries and the child is alert and crying. You determine that you need to immobilize the patient in the seat.

Pediatric Immobilization Station Scenario C

[To be read aloud to the group]

You are dispatched to the scene of a single motor vehicle crash. The vehicle left the gravel road and rolled over several times in the ditch. The occupants of the vehicle, a mother and her 10-month-old child, were ejected on the first rollover. Your unit is assigned the infant. You find the infant still in the car-seat restraint device lying face down in the ditch. The child is crying loudly, and you cannot see the patient to perform any type of assessment. You determine that the child will have to be turned over to complete any assessment and to immobilize.

Immobilization Technique—Pediatric Patients Not in a Car-Seat Style Restraint Device

1. Apply and maintain manual stabilization with neutral alignment
   Measure and apply cervical collar
   Apply short board if indicated
   Move patient onto long backboard
   Pad behind the patient's shoulders and spine to maintain neutral alignment
2. Secure to board
   a. Torso
      Pelvis
      Lower extremities
      Head

Equipment List for Pediatric Immobilization Scenarios D, E, and F

1. Blankets and towels
2. Cervical collars (pediatric)
3. Patient
4. Spinal immobilization equipment (pediatric)
5. Straps
6. Tape

Pediatric Immobilization Scenario D

[To be read aloud to the group]

Your service is dispatched to the scene of a single motor vehicle crash on a gravel road. Upon arrival, you find an older sport utility vehicle that has rolled over. All the occupants have been ejected. Your patient is a 7-year-old lying prone in the roadway with the hands above the head. The patient is nonresponsive with a patent airway and adequate ventilations. You determine that the patient must be turned and secured with spinal immobilization.

Pediatric Immobilization Scenario E

[To be read aloud to the group]

Your service is dispatched to the local softball diamond for a child who fell from the bleachers. Upon arrival, you are directed behind the bleachers for an 8-year-old who fell from the top of the bleachers while cheering for a brother's ball team. The patient's mother states the child has no past medical history and is taking no medications. You find the patient lying supine on the ground, conscious and alert. The patient states not being able to move the legs and that it "hurts real bad" in the lower back. Your assessment confirms the patient's complaints.

Pediatric Immobilization Scenario F

[To be read aloud to the group]

Your service is dispatched to the scene of a single vehicle crash. The driver of the vehicle lost control and slid sideways into a tree. The car sustained major damage on the passenger's side, and access can only be obtained from the driver's side. The driver has been removed from the car, and the passenger now must be removed. After assessment, you determine that the 8-year-old passenger has no major injuries, but you feel that immobilization is needed before moving this patient.

SPINAL IMMOBILIZATION SKILLS STATION

INTRODUCTION

Spinal immobilization is a vital skill for all levels of prehospital providers when treating a trauma patient. This skill may include techniques ranging from simple manual stabilization to complete immobilization to a long backboard. Improper immobilization techniques may cause the trauma patient to suffer from an unnecessary spinal injury. Each trauma patient must be assessed for any suspected spinal injury and be properly immobilized based on the assessment and/or mechanism of injury. Mastery of spinal immobilization techniques is necessary for all prehospital care providers.

The teaching of skills within this station in no way implies that the provider will be able to perform the skills outside of the classroom arena. All participants must understand that skills discussed, viewed, and/or practiced within this teaching station may only be performed in a nonclassroom situation when authorized by their certifying or licensing agency.

Equipment List

Item	Quantity
Blankets/sheets	4
Cervical collars	Multiple sizes
Long backboard	1
Motorcycle helmet	1
Scoop-style stretcher	1
Short backboard	1
Straps	6
Towels	4

EVALUATOR INSTRUCTIONS

Give a demonstration/overview of each procedure that follows and answer any questions the participants may have regarding the procedures. After demonstration, allow supervised practice of each procedure with individual help as needed.

Participants should perform skills while observing proper body substance isolation and performing other proper safety/performance techniques. Verbalization of performance by the participants will not be acceptable practice.

Participants need only demonstrate those procedures that are within their scope of practice. Participants may choose to demonstrate procedures that are outside of their scope of practice. Participants with limited scope of practice must understand that any procedure observed, practiced, and/or demonstrated by them within this station does not allow them to perform the procedure in a nonclassroom setting without approval of their certifying or licensing agency.

Refer to the fourth edition of *Prehospital Trauma Life Support* (the PHTLS provider textbook), Chapter 10: Spine Management Skills, for sequenced steps for each procedure.

SPINAL IMMOBILIZATION PROCEDURES

Manual Stabilization and Neutral Alignment of the Head and Neck Techniques (Basic and Advanced Providers)

Objectives
At the completion of this skill station, the participants will be able to:
1. Identify indications and contraindications for the use of manual stabilization and neutral alignment of the head and neck techniques
2. Demonstrate the manual techniques of stabilization and neutral alignment of the patient's head and neck

Demonstrated Skills by the Participants:
1. Manual technique of stabilization and neutral alignment of the patient's head and neck from in front of the patient (sitting and standing patients)
2. Manual technique of stabilization and neutral alignment of the patient's head and neck from behind the patient (sitting and standing patients)
3. Manual technique of stabilization and neutral alignment of the patient's head and neck from the side of the patient (sitting, standing, and lying patients)
4. Manual technique of stabilization and neutral alignment of the patient's head and neck from above the patient (lying patient)

Sizing and Application of Cervical Collar Techniques (Basic and Advanced Providers)

Objectives
At the completion of this skill station, the participants will be able to:
1. Identify indications and contraindications for the use of a cervical collar
2. Demonstrate an approved method of sizing and selecting a cervical collar, according to manufacturer's recommendations, while manual stabilization is maintained
3. Demonstrate proper application and securing of a properly sized cervical collar, according to manufacturer's recommendations, while manual stabilization is maintained

Demonstrated Skills by the Participants:
1. Sizing and selecting a cervical collar while manual stabilization is maintained
2. Application and securing of a properly sized cervical collar while manual stabilization is maintained

Standing Backboard Techniques
(Basic and Advanced Providers)

Objectives
At the completion of this skill station, the participants will be able to:
1. Identify indications and contraindications for the application of a standing backboard
2. Demonstrate an approved method of providing spinal immobilization to a standing patient

Demonstrated Skill by the Participants:
1. Spinal immobilization of a standing patient

Transfer of a Lying Patient to a Long Backboard
(Basic and Advanced Providers)

Objectives
At the completion of this skill station, the participants will be able to:
1. Identify indications and contraindications for the transfer of a lying patient to a long backboard
2. Demonstrate a proper technique to transfer a lying (supine and prone) trauma patient to a long backboard
3. Demonstrate proper use of padding and buttress material to fill all voids when securing a patient to a long backboard
4. Demonstrate securing a patient to a long backboard

Demonstrated Skills by the Participants:
1. Transfer of a supine patient to a long backboard (logroll and scoop stretcher)
2. Transfer of a prone patient to a long backboard
3. Use of padding and buttress material to fill all identified voids
4. Securing of a trauma patient to a long backboard

Helmet Removal (Basic Providers)

Objectives
At the completion of this skill station, the participants will be able to:
1. Identify indications and contraindications for the removal of a helmet
2. Demonstrate proper removal of a helmet while maintaining manual stabilization and neutral alignment of the trauma patient's head and neck

Demonstrated Skill by the Participants:
1. Removal of a helmet while maintaining manual stabilization and neutral alignment of the patient's head and neck

IMPROVED LOGROLL
TO LONG BACKBOARD

Technique
A. Provider #1 obtains manual stabilization of the patient's head and neck from above the patient's head.
B. Provider #2 measures and applies a cervical collar.
C. Provider #4 positions a long backboard alongside the patient.

D. Providers #2 and #3 examine and then place the patient's extremities into an in-line anatomic position.
E. Provider #2 assumes a position at the patient's chest, opposite side from the backboard.
F. Provider #3 assumes a position at the patient's upper legs, opposite side from the backboard.
G. Provider #3 gathers the patient's cuffs to the patient's pants or holds the patient's ankles with the feet and legs in a neutral position with the hand closest to the patient's feet, and places the other hand on the opposite side of the patient under the hip area.
H. Provider #2 places his or her hand closest to the patient's head, under the patient's shoulder on the side opposite of the provider.
I. Provider #2's hand closest to the patient's feet is placed under the patient's hip on the side opposite of the provider and closer to the patient's feet than provider #3's hand.
J. Provider #1 will control the turning of the patient onto his or her side in a unified movement.
K. Provider #4 will slide the long backboard under the patient with the foot end of the board placed at the level of the patient's knees.
L. On command from provider #1, the patient is rolled down onto the backboard. The patient should not be slid sideways onto the board.
M. Provider #2 places his or her hands in the patient's axilla (arm pit) area.
N. Provider #3 places his or her hands on each side of the patient's pelvis at the hips.
O. On command from provider #1, the patient is moved upward and placed in the center of the backboard.
P. The patient is then secured to the long backboard with appropriate padding (torso, pelvis, lower extremities, and then head).

RAPID EXTRICATION SKILLS STATION

INTRODUCTION

Rapid extrication involves removing a trauma patient from an automobile while maintaining minimal spinal stabilization without the use of traditional immobilization equipment. This technique is accomplished through the use of manual stabilization and a team approach. Although this technique cannot be used in every situation or every make of automobile, the basic principles can be applied. Rapid extrication should only be used when the patient has been assessed as having a life-threatening condition or when a hazardous situation exists where the patient must be moved immediately. At all other times, the trauma patient should be immobilized and moved only after the application of standard spinal immobilization techniques.

The teaching of skills within this station in no way implies that the provider will be able to perform the skills outside of the classroom arena. All participants must understand that skills discussed, viewed, and/or practiced within this teaching station may only be performed in a nonclassroom situation when authorized by their certifying or licensing agency.

Equipment List

Item	Quantity
Automobile (four-door preferred)	1
Cervical collars	Multiple sizes
Cot (optional)	1
Long backboard	1
Patient	1
Stethoscope	1
Straps	6

EVALUATOR INSTRUCTIONS

Give a demonstration/overview of each procedure that follows and answer any questions the participants may have regarding the procedures. After demonstration, allow supervised practice of each procedure with individual help as needed.

Participants should perform skills while observing proper body substance isolation and performing other proper safety/performance techniques. Verbalization of performance by the participants will not be acceptable practice.

Participants need only demonstrate those procedures that are within their scope of practice. Participants may choose to demonstrate procedures that are outside of their scope of practice. Participants with limited scope of practice must understand that any procedure observed, practiced, and/or demonstrated by them within this station does not allow them to perform the procedure in a nonclassroom setting without approval of their certifying or licensing agency.

Refer to the fourth edition of the PHTLS provider textbook, Chapter 10: Spine Management Skills, to find sequenced steps for each procedure.

RAPID EXTRICATION PROCEDURES

Rapid Extrication (Basic and Advanced Providers)

Objectives
At the completion of this skill station, the participants will be able to:
1. Identify the indications and contraindications for the use of rapid extrication
2. Demonstrate the proper technique for rapid extrication while maintaining minimal spinal immobilization

Demonstrated Skills by the Participants:
1. Rapid extrication of a trauma patient while maintaining minimal spinal immobilization
2. Assume and demonstrate each team member's role during rapid extrication

FINAL EVALUATION STATIONS

INTRODUCTION

The stations included here are for the final evaluation process. There are three final scenario stations that each group must complete. Scenarios and evaluation flow sheets are provided for each station. (See Section V for the *Final Evaluation Station Scenario Flow Sheet.*) Each group need only successfully complete one scenario for each station. Evaluators for each final station ideally will be individuals who have successfully completed the PHTLS Instructor Program. Leadership of the group should change for each final evaluation station to allow all participants to experience the responsibility of managing a trauma patient. Each group of participants should be evaluated on their combined efforts to effectively assess and treat a trauma patient in the provided scenarios. Evaluation of each station is based on current acceptable practices of assessment and treatment of a trauma patient. Each group will either successfully or unsuccessfully complete the scenario as a whole. Debriefing of the group as a whole after completing the station is recommended. If a group is unsuccessful during the final evaluation process, remediation of the identified difficulties should occur, and the group should be offered another opportunity to successfully complete the failed station. In the event that a group is unsuccessful on the second attempt of any failed station, plans should be made for the group to attend and complete another entire PHTLS program.

EVALUATOR INSTRUCTIONS

Identify which scenario will be used for your final evaluation station from the choices contained within this section of the *Instructor Manual.* Only the scenarios provided within this section of the *Instructor Manual* may be used for the final evaluation process. Each scenario contains an evaluation scenario, equipment list, patient instructions, participant's instructions, and an evaluation flow sheet. Assemble all the required equipment, instruct the patient on his or her role, and moulage the patient according to the injuries for the selected scenario. When the station and patient are prepared, assemble the group to be evaluated, read to them the participant's instructions, and answer any questions pertaining to the scenario. After answering any questions, identify who will be the leader of the group for this station. Identifying the group leader will give you a single person on which to focus your attention, yet each participant is expected to contribute to the assessment and treatment of the patient. Allow the group an opportunity to review their equipment and request any additional equipment not present. When the group is ready, read the scenario aloud and ask if they understand the scenario or have any questions. If there are no questions or after answering any questions, begin the evaluation process. Chart the process of the group on the scenario flow sheet. If the group is not assessing or treating the patient correctly, you may wish to worsen the patient's condition as necessary. When the group has completed the scenario or after a total time of 10 minutes has elapsed of assessing and treating the patient, end the scenario and debrief the group as a whole. After debriefing the group, direct them back to the program coordinator for their next assignment. Prepare the scene and patient for the next group.

PARTICIPANT INSTRUCTIONS

[To be read aloud to the group]

You will be dispatched as a group to the scene of a trauma patient. You will need to assess and treat the patient according to your findings. You will be evaluated as a group, not by individual performance. Please identify one person at this time to serve as your group leader for this scenario. My primary attention will be given to this individual. Direct all assessment and treatment toward your group leader in such a fashion that I am aware of your performances. The role of group leader will change for each scenario. You will have a maximum of 10 minutes to complete this scenario. Please perform procedures as you would in a real situation. You may wish to verbalize your performance as you complete each step for the purpose of evaluation. All invasive procedures should be verbalized and not actually performed on the patient. Please review all your equipment before beginning the scenario at this time.

    Do you understand what is expected of you as a group?

    Do you have any questions?

    Are you ready for your dispatch information?

FINAL EVALUATION STATION I

FINAL EVALUATION SCENARIO IA

Evaluator Information

The group will be dispatched to the scene of a single motor vehicle crash. The patient was driving home after attending a wedding rehearsal dinner party in the early evening hours on a warm Friday night. The patient apparently lost control of the car on a suburban street, striking a large tree head-on. The group will find a single, nonrestrained 20- to 30-year-old patient, the driver of the automobile, slumped over the steering wheel and responsive to verbal stimulus. The windows of the vehicle are open, and the doors are unlocked. Injuries will include bruising with a small laceration and no active bleeding to the right frontal area of the head. Bruising will be found over the midchest area and abdomen from the steering wheel. The patient will not have a palpable radial pulse, but will have a weak, rapid carotid pulse (over 110). Skin will be pale in color and cool and damp to the touch. Respirations are rapid and shallow, and the patient can only speak in short two- to three-word statements with shortness of breath. There are diminished sounds on the patient's right chest area when the group auscultates for breathing. The patient will complain of pain and tenderness upon palpation of the chest and abdomen area. No other injuries or complaints will be found. No significant past medical history, allergies, or current medications will be noted.

Equipment List for Scenario IA

1. Automobile
2. Blankets and towels
3. Blood pressure equipment
4. Body substance protection equipment
5. Cervical collars
6. IV equipment

7. Medic box
8. Moulaged patient
9. Needle decompression equipment
10. PASG
11. Spinal immobilization equipment
12. Stethoscope
13. Straps
14. Supplemental oxygen equipment
15. Tape

Patient Instructions for Scenario IA

You are the patient in a single vehicle crash who lost control of the auto and struck a tree head-on in a residential area. Your injuries are described as follows. Please act according to the scenario and injuries and repeat the same performance for each group. Based on the assessment and treatment rendered by each group, your condition will either stabilize or worsen. Please pay attention to the evaluator for signals on changes in your condition. At the completion of each scenario, the evaluator may ask for your input on the group's performance. Please supply the evaluator with the requested information from an objective viewpoint. The evaluator will have the final say on the group's overall performance.

Moulaged Injuries for Scenario IA

Body Area/Function	Injury/Response
Head/face	Bruise, small laceration on right forehead
	No active bleeding
Chest/abdomen	Steering wheel bruising
	Pain and tenderness upon palpation
	Diminished breath sounds on right side
Level of consciousness	Responsive to verbal stimulus
Breathing	Rapid, shallow respirations
	Short two- to three-word statements; SOB
Circulation	No palpable radial pulse
	Rapid, weak carotid pulse
	No external hemorrhage
Skin	Pale
	Cool and damp to touch
Extremities	No injuries
	Free movement
History	No past medical history
	No allergies
	No current medications
	Ate a full meal after rehearsal
	Consumed three to four mixed drinks with dinner

Proper Treatment of Scenario IA

1. Complete initial (primary) assessment
2. Identify critical patient (chest/abdomen injuries)
3. Perform rapid extrication
4. Establish and maintain manual stabilization of head and neck until the head is secured to a backboard

5. Properly size, select, apply, and secure cervical collar
6. Transfer of patient to a long backboard while maintaining minimal spinal immobilization
7. Timely transport of patient to an appropriate level trauma facility
8. Application of high-flow oxygen en route (may be done on-scene)
9. Needle decompression of right chest (if skill is within the participant's scope of practice) en route
10. Consider the use of PASG
11. Consider the initiation of IV(s) en route (if skill is within the participant's scope of practice)
12. Reassessment of patient's condition

Dispatch Information for Scenario IA

[To be read aloud to the group]

Your ambulance service is dispatched to the scene of a single vehicle crash. The car struck a tree head-on in a residential neighborhood. It is in the late evening hours on a clear, warm, summer Friday evening. Law enforcement is on the scene directing traffic and is willing to help with reasonable requests.

Do you have any questions before beginning?

Please begin; your time starts now!

FINAL EVALUATION SCENARIO IB —————

Evaluator Information

The group will be dispatched to the scene of a single vehicle rollover. The patient was driving from town to a rural home when the right front tire dropped off the shoulder of the gravel road and rolled the vehicle over sideways one complete revolution. The car came to rest upright on its wheels in the ditch. It is a clear, warm, summer day. The local volunteer fire service arrived at the scene just before the ambulance service and is willing to direct traffic and help with manpower when requested. The patient is a 30- to 40-year-old individual found sitting upright on the driver's side of the car, leaning against the door, with the head resting against the shoulder. Shoulder and lap restraints were not in use. The front windshield is cracked, but intact. The side windows of the car are down, and all doors are unlocked and can be opened by hand. The scene will be safe for the providers. Patient injuries will include a large scalp laceration with minimal bleeding on the upper part of the head. There are multiple small cuts and abrasions to the left arm, again with minimal venous bleeding. The patient will be nonresponsive to both verbal and painful stimulus. Respirations are ataxic and sonorous between 8 to 14 per minute. Blood-tinged drainage appears from the left ear opening. The patient will have a slow, weak, radial pulse of 48. If the pupils are checked, the providers will find the right pupil fixed and dilated. No history, allergy, or medication information is available. No other injuries will be found.

Equipment List for Scenario IB

1. Automobile
2. Blankets and towels
3. Blood pressure equipment
4. Body substance protection equipment
5. Cervical collars

6. IV equipment
7. Medic response box
8. Moulaged patient
9. PASG
10. Spinal immobilization equipment
11. Stethoscope
12. Straps
13. Supplemental oxygen equipment
14. Tape

Patient Instructions for Scenario IB

You are the patient of a single vehicle rollover. Your injuries are described as follows. Please act according to the scenario and injuries and repeat the same performance for each group. Based on the assessment and treatment rendered by each group, your condition will either stabilize or worsen. Please pay attention to the evaluator for signals on changes to your condition. At the completion of each scenario, the evaluator may ask for your input on the group's performance. Please supply the evaluator with the requested information from an objective viewpoint. The evaluator will have the final say on the group's overall performance.

Moulaged Injuries for Scenario IB

Body/Area	Injury/Response
Head/face	Large open laceration to superior portion of the head with minimal active bleeding
	Blood-tinged drainage from the left ear opening
	Fixed and dilated right pupil
Chest/abdomen	No injuries
Extremities	Multiple small lacerations and abrasions to the left arm; minimal venous bleeding
Level of consciousness	Nonresponsive to verbal or painful stimulus
Breathing	Ataxic and sonorous; 8–14/minute
Circulation	Slow, weak radial pulse (48)
	No external hemorrhage
Skin	Pale in color
	Warm and moist to the touch
	Delayed capillary refill
History	None available

Proper Treatment of Scenario IB

1. Complete initial (primary) assessment
2. Identify critical patient (head injury)
3. Perform rapid extrication
4. Establish and maintain manual stabilization of head and neck until the head is secured to a backboard
5. Properly size, select, apply, and secure cervical collar
6. Transfer of patient to a long backboard while maintaining minimal spinal immobilization
7. Timely transport of patient to an appropriate level trauma facility
8. Application of high-flow oxygen and assisted ventilations en route (may be done on-scene)

9. Loose dressing and bandage of head wound
10. Consider the use of PASG
11. Consider the initiation of IV(s) en route (if skill is within the participant's scope of practice)
12. Consider intubation (if skill is within the participant's scope of practice)
13. Consider hyperventilation
14. Consider a head elevated transport position while maintaining spinal immobilization
15. Reassessment of patient's condition

Dispatch Information for Scenario IB

[To be read aloud to the group]

Your ambulance service is dispatched to the scene of a single vehicle rollover. The car went off the shoulder of the gravel road and rolled over sideways one complete revolution. The car is sitting upright on its wheel in the ditch. It is in the daylight hours of a warm summer day. The local volunteer fire department arrived at the scene just before you and is willing to help with reasonable requests.

Do you have any questions before beginning?

Please begin; your time starts now!

FINAL EVALUATION STATION II

FINAL EVALUATION SCENARIO IIA

Evaluator Information

The group will be dispatched to the home of an elderly person (late 60s) who fell down while walking up the sidewalk near home to water the flowers. The slightly obese patient will be sitting on the sidewalk and leaning back on the elbows for comfort. A neighbor who witnessed the fall was in attendance but left after the ambulance's arrival. The patient will be conscious and alert and complaining of pain in the right hip area. The patient tripped on a raised portion of the sidewalk. The right leg/foot will be externally rotated and shortened. Abrasions are on the palm surface of both hands from the fall. The patient has a past medical history of COPD, ASHD, hypertension, diabetes, and angina and is currently taking the following medications: Lasix, nitroglycerin, insulin, digitalis, stool softener, and ASA. The patient has no known allergies. The patient resides alone at the home where the fall happened. Respirations are 26/minute with pursed-lip exhalation. Redness and edema are noted in both ankles. Skin is red, warm, and damp to the touch. The radial pulse is 132/minute and irregular. Lung sounds are equal and wet on both sides upon auscultation. No other injuries will be noted.

Equipment List for Scenario IIA

1. Blankets and towels
2. Blood pressure equipment
3. Body substance protection equipment
4. Cervical collars

5. IV equipment
6. Medic response kit
7. Moulaged patient
8. Spinal immobilization equipment
9. Stethoscope
10. Straps
11. Supplemental oxygen equipment
12. Tape

Patient Instructions for Scenario IIA

You are the slightly obese patient who fell outside at home. You tripped over a raised portion of the sidewalk while you were out watering your flowers. Your injuries are described as follows. Please act according to the scenario and injuries and repeat the same performance for each group. Based on the assessment and treatment rendered by each group, your condition will either stabilize or worsen. Please pay attention to the evaluator for signals on changes to your condition. At the completion of each scenario, the evaluator may ask for your input on the group's performance. Please supply the evaluator with the requested information from an objective viewpoint. The evaluator will have the final say on the group's overall performance.

Moulaged Injuries for Scenario IIA

Body/Area	Injury/Response
Head/face	No injuries
Chest/abdomen	No injuries
	Equal and wet lung sounds upon auscultation
Extremities	Abrasions on palm surface of both hands
	Pain in both hands and shoulders upon examination (from fall)
	External rotation and shortening of right leg
	Redness and edema in both ankles
	Pain in right hip area upon palpation
Level of consciousness	Alert and conscious
	States they "should of fixed that darn old sidewalk years ago"
Respirations	26/minute
	Pursed-lip exhalations
Circulation	Rapid, irregular radial pulse (132)
Skin	Red in color
	Warm and moist
History	Diabetic, COPD, ASHD, hypertension, angina
	No known allergies
	Medications of Lasix, nitroglycerin, ASA, insulin, and stool softener
	Low-flow oxygen (PRN)

Proper Treatment of Scenario IIA

1. Complete initial (primary) assessment
2. Identify noncritical patient (fractured hip)
3. Complete detailed (secondary) assessment

4. Immobilization of the right hip and leg
5. Transfer to long backboard
6. Transfer to nearest facility
7. Consider supplemental oxygen (low flow)
8. Supportive treatment en route

Dispatch Information for Scenario IIA

[To be read aloud to the group]

Your service is dispatched to the scene of an elderly patient who fell outside at home. The neighbor who witnessed the fall left upon your arrival. It is a clear sunny midmorning.

Do you have any questions before beginning?

Please begin; your time starts now!

FINAL EVALUATION SCENARIO IIB

Evaluator Information

The group will be dispatched to the scene of a bicycle crash on one of the local bicycle trails. The patient will be a 19- to 22-year-old college person who was on the way to class when the front wheel of the bicycle fell off the pathway, throwing the patient from the bicycle. The patient will be found sitting under one of the trees and holding the right arm against the chest and supported in the lap. There are a couple of other students in attendance. It is a warm and sunny weekday afternoon. The patient will be conscious and alert. The only complaints will be pain in the patient's right elbow and right ankle area. There is increased pain with any attempt to move either extremity. Deformities are found in the right elbow and right ankle. Abrasions are found on the patient's right forearm, shoulder, right buttock, and lower leg. The patient was wearing a helmet, but it is now removed. There will be no significant past history, no known allergies, and no current medications being taken.

Equipment List for Scenario IIB

1. Bicycle and helmet
2. Blankets and towels
3. Blood pressure equipment
4. Body substance protection equipment
5. Cervical collars
6. IV equipment
7. Medic response box
8. Moulaged patient
9. Spinal immobilization equipment
10. Splints
11. Stethoscope
12. Straps
13. Supplemental oxygen equipment
14. Tape

Patient Instructions for Scenario IIB

You are the patient of a single bicycle crash. You were riding to class when the front wheel of your bicycle fell off the pathway and threw you from your bike. You were wearing a helmet at the time of the crash and removed it afterward. Your injuries are described as follows. Please act according to the scenario and injuries and repeat the same performance for each group. Based on the assessment and treatment rendered by each group, your condition will either stabilize or worsen. Please pay attention to the evaluator for signals on changes to your condition. At the completion of each scenario, the evaluator may ask for your input on the group's performance. Please supply the evaluator with the requested information from an objective viewpoint. The evaluator will have the final say on the group's overall performance.

Moulaged Injuries for Scenario IIB

Body Area/Function	Injury/Response
Head/face	No injuries
Chest/abdomen/back	No injuries
Extremities	Abrasions to right shoulder, right buttock, right leg
	Deformity of right elbow and right ankle
	Increased pain with any movement of the right extremities
Skin	Pink in color
	Dry and warm
Level of consciousness	Alert and conscious
	Appropriate answers
Breathing	Regular, 18/minute
Breath sounds	Clear and equal
History	No significant history

Proper Treatment for Scenario IIB

1. Complete initial (primary) assessment
2. Identify noncritical patient (fractured wrist and ankle)
3. Complete detailed (secondary) assessment
4. Splint both suspected fractures
5. Transfer to a long backboard and secure
6. Reassess patient's condition
7. Transfer to nearest facility

Dispatch Information for Scenario IIB

[To be read aloud to the group]

Your service is dispatched to the bicycle paths in the local college area. A single rider lost control of the bicycle and suffered a fall. Two other students are in attendance upon your arrival. It is a warm, sunny, weekday afternoon.

Do you have any questions before beginning?

Please begin; your time starts now!

FINAL EVALUATION STATION III

FINAL EVALUATION SCENARIO IIIA

Evaluator Information

The group will be dispatched to the scene of a young male in his early 20s. The patient will be found wearing dirty clothing and lying on the sofa of his home. He will be conscious and somewhat alert, easily responding to verbal commands, and unable to sit up or stand without feeling like he is going to pass out. It is midmorning (around 10:00 am) on Sunday. The patient states that he "really tied one on" last night at the local bar. While walking home around 1:30 am this morning, he was beaten up and robbed by a gang of teenagers. The gang members hit him in the abdomen a couple of times with a baseball bat and pummeled him with their fists when he refused to give them his money. The patient's face will show signs of a fistfight, swelling and bruising around the eyes, laceration to the lower lip without active bleeding, and dried blood around both nares. The patient's left chest and abdomen areas are bruised, and he will complain of pain only upon palpation. Minor abrasions will be noted on the patient's knuckles of both hands. There will be a long-standing history of severe alcohol dependence and abuse but no other significant history, no known allergies, and currently no medications being taken.

Equipment List for Scenario IIIA

1. Moulaged patient
2. Medic response box
3. Stethoscope
4. Blood pressure equipment
5. Supplemental oxygen equipment
6. Cervical collars
7. Spinal immobilization equipment
8. Straps
9. Tape
10. Blankets and towels
11. IV equipment
12. PASG
13. Body substance protection equipment

Patient Instructions for Scenario IIIA

You are a male patient in your early 20s who called for the ambulance because when you attempted to stand up or sit up you would almost pass out. You were out drinking last night (Saturday) from around 5:00 pm until approximately 1:15 am this morning. On your way home, a gang of teenagers (five to seven) had approached you. A couple of the gang members told you to give them all your money or they would have to hurt you. You refused to give them your money, and an altercation began. One of the members hit you a couple times with a baseball bat in the chest and belly. The other members hit you repeatedly with their fists. You managed to hit a couple of the members with your fists, but to no avail. After knocking you to the ground, they took your money and ran away. You got up and finished walking home, where you laid down on the sofa and slept until around 10:00 Sunday morning. You attempted to get off the sofa, but when you sat up you got dizzy. After sitting there for a few minutes, you attempted to stand up and nearly passed out. You tried a couple more times with the same results. You called for the ambulance and laid back down on the sofa waiting for their arrival. You are able to respond to their questions slowly, and you keep closing your eyes because you are tired. Your injuries are described as follows. Please act according to the scenario and injuries and repeat the same performance for each group. Based on the assessment and treatment rendered by each group, your condition will either stabilize or worsen. Please pay attention to the evaluator for signals on changes to your condition. At the completion of each scenario, the evaluator may ask for your input on the group's performance. Please supply the evaluator with the requested information from an objective viewpoint. The evaluator will have the final say on the group's overall performance.

Moulaged Injuries for Scenario IIIA

Body Area/Function	Injury/Response
Head/face	Swelling, bruising, tenderness around both eyes
	Laceration on the lower lip without active bleeding
	Dried blood around both nares
Chest/abdomen	Bruising to the left chest and upper abdomen areas
	Pain upon palpation
Level of consciousness	Responds to verbal stimulus slowly
	Tries to keep eyes closed whenever not responding to a question—Tired
Breathing	22/minute
Breath sounds	Clear and equal
Circulation	Weak, rapid radial pulse (128)
	Delayed capillary refill when tested
Skin	Pink in color
	Warm and damp
Extremities	Minor abrasions on both sets of knuckles
History	Long-standing dependence and abuse of alcohol
	States: "really tied one on" last night
	Ingestion of a greater then normal amount of beer and liquor last night
	Last meal yesterday at lunch time

Proper Treatment of Scenario IIIA

1. Complete initial (primary) assessment
2. Identify critical patient (suspected internal bleeding)
3. Rapid assessment for other underlying injuries
4. Decision for timely transport
5. Selection of appropriate facility (surgery capabilities)
6. Apply high-flow supplemental oxygen
7. Consider application of PASG en route
8. Consider initiation of IV(s) en route (if skill is within the participant's scope of practice)

9. Interaction with medical control as necessary
10. Detailed assessment performed en route if time and resources allow

Dispatch Information for Scenario IIIA

[To be read aloud to the group]

Your service is dispatched to the home of a young male patient who feels like he is going to pass out each time he attempts to sit or stand. Upon arrival you find the front door unlocked, and the patient yells at you to come on in.

Do you have any questions before beginning?

Please begin; your time starts now!

FINAL EVALUATION SCENARIO IIIB

Evaluator Information

The group will be dispatched to the scene of a patient who fell yesterday and now has a lot of pain. The patient was coming downstairs from the bedroom yesterday morning, fell down about eight stairs, and landed at the bottom of the stairway. The patient was able to get up and go about normal activities. At around 8:00 pm last night, the patient started experiencing some chest and right shoulder discomfort. The patient took some Tylenol #3 that was available at home from a previous injury and that helped with the pain. This morning the patient was unable to go to work because of the pain. Now there are complaints of pain in the right chest and right shoulder, along with some numbness and tingling in both of the upper extremities. The patient has taken three of the Tylenol #3 today to help control the pain without success. It is now 2:00 pm in the afternoon, and the patient meets the crew at the door and will stand and talk to them at all times. During assessment the group will find decreased breath sounds on the right chest area and decreased use of both upper extremities due to the numbness and tingling. There is no other significant past history, no known allergies, and no other medications taken other than the Tylenol #3.

Equipment List for Scenario IIIB

1. Blankets and towels
2. Blood pressure equipment
3. Body substance protection equipment
4. Cervical collars
5. IV equipment
6. Medic response box
7. Moulaged patient
8. Needle decompression equipment
9. PASG
10. Spinal immobilization equipment
11. Stethoscope
12. Straps
13. Supplemental oxygen equipment
14. Tape

Patient Instructions for Scenario IIIB

You will be portraying a patient who fell down the stairs at home yesterday morning while coming downstairs from your bedroom. You fell down approximately eight stairs and landed at the bottom without losing consciousness. You were able to go about your daily activities without problems. Around 8:00 pm last night you started to experience pain and discomfort in your right chest area and right shoulder area. You took a couple of Tylenol #3 you had at home from an old knee injury. This initially helped with the pain, and you were able to go to bed. This morning you woke up with increased pain in your chest and shoulder and also numbness and tingling in both of your upper extremities with some loss of motion/control. You took three more of the Tylenol #3, but this did not seem to help. The pain increased enough this afternoon that you felt you had to see someone. Your injuries and responses are described as follows. Please act according to the scenario and injuries and repeat the same performance for each group. Based on the assessment and treatment rendered by each group, your condition will either stabilize or worsen. Please pay attention to the evaluator for signals on changes to your condition. At the completion of each scenario, the evaluator may ask for your input on the group's performance. Please supply the evaluator with the requested information from an objective viewpoint. The evaluator will have the final say on the group's overall performance.

Moulaged Injuries for Scenario IIIB

Body Area/Function	Injury/Response
Head/face	No injuries
Chest/abdomen	Bruising/ecchymosis on right upper chest, shoulder, right side of lower cervical area
Extremities	Numbness and tingling in both upper extremities
	Slight loss of control/function
Skin	Dusky in color
	Warm and moist
Level of consciousness	Alert and responsive
Breathing	28 and shallow
	Hurts to breathe deep
Breath sounds	Decreased on right side
Circulation/blood pressure	Radial pulse (118)
	BP: 134/76
History	No significant past history
	Tylenol #3

Proper Treatment of Scenario IIIB

1. Complete initial (primary) survey
2. Identify critical patient (pneumothorax, suspected spinal injury)
3. Rapid assessment for other injuries
4. Spinal immobilization (standing backboard)
5. Decision for timely transport
6. Selection of appropriate facility
7. Apply high-flow oxygen

8. Consider decompression of right-side pneumothorax (if skill is within the participant's scope of practice)
9. Consider initiation of IV en route (if skill is within the participant's scope of practice)
10. Interaction with medical control as necessary
11. Detailed (secondary) assessment performed en route if time and resources allow

Dispatch Information for Scenario IIIB

[To be read aloud to the group]

Your service is dispatched to the home of a patient (mid-30s) who complains of pain and discomfort in the right chest and shoulder from a fall yesterday. The patient will meet you at the door. It is approximately 2:00 pm in the afternoon.

Do you have any questions before beginning?

Please begin; your time starts now!

SECTION III

Instructor Program

PHTLS INSTRUCTOR PROGRAM

INTRODUCTION

Goal

The program goal is to provide the PHTLS instructor/coordinator candidate with the knowledge, skills, and support materials necessary to conduct and/or participate as faculty in any approved PHTLS course.

Setting

The program is ideally conducted in conjunction with a PHTLS provider course. Depending on the target audience, the instructor portion of the course may be taken before or after a provider course.

Time

The instructor/coordinator workshop consists of lectures and practical skills stations that can be completed in a time period of approximately 8 hours. This time frame may be altered as necessary to ensure that the participants have completed and/or met all the stated objectives.

Materials

Each instructor/coordinator candidate should have a copy of the current PHTLS provider textbook, the *PHTLS Instructor Manual,* and evaluation materials.

Instructors

Each program shall be conducted with at least one PHTLS national or affiliate faculty member present. The total number of faculty will be determined by the number of participating instructor candidates and at the discretion of the national faculty representative.

Instructor/Coordinator Candidates

Each instructor/coordinator candidate will have completed, at a minimum, a PHTLS provider course or a PHTLS refresher course within the last 3 years. Individuals may also be given provider status by having successfully completed a BTLS provider course and a PHTLS refresher course.

For admission to the instructor/coordinator workshop, each candidate must present a letter of recommendation to the instructor/coordinator workshop's course coordinator, from the coordinator of the provider course he or she attended, or from any other PHTLS national or affiliate faculty.

Objectives

At the completion of the instructor/coordinator workshop, each participant will be able to:
1. Identify the components of the PHTLS organizational structure.
2. Identify members of the PHTLS executive council.
3. Identify each of the PHTLS regions.

4. Identify the PHTLS state and regional coordinators particular to the participant's course site.
5. Access the international PHTLS office by phone, fax, E-mail, and Web site.
6. Complete the precourse and postcourse paperwork necessary to conduct a PHTLS provider course.
7. Identify each of the PHTLS courses.
8. Identify the objectives a participant must meet to successfully complete a PHTLS provider course.
9. Assemble each teaching and final assessment station.
10. Explain the answer for each question on the precourse and postcourse written evaluation.

INSTRUCTOR/COORDINATOR WORKSHOP

SCHEDULE

Subject	Time Frame
Welcome, Registration, and Introductions	15 minutes
Administrative Overview	90 minutes
Break	15 minutes
Teaching Techniques	60 minutes
Lunch	60 minutes
Teaching Stations Overview	150 minutes
Break	15 minutes
Final Assessment Stations Overview	60 minutes
Written Evaluation Overview	30 minutes
Summary	15 minutes

Welcome, Registration, and Introductions

Participants should complete all registration forms and other related items during this time. Letters of recommendation and copies of provider and refresher program recognition can also be gathered at this time.

Administrative Overview

During the administrative overview, the following should be covered:
1. PHTLS organizational structure
2. PHTLS executive council members
3. NAEMT and ACS/COT affiliation
4. PHTLS regions
5. PHTLS staff directory
6. Precourse paperwork
7. Postcourse paperwork
8. PHTLS International Office and support material

Teaching Techniques

This lecture will discuss techniques needed to help both new and seasoned instructors deliver the PHTLS materials in a more effective manner.

Teaching Stations Overview

This section is designed to be completed in four 45-minute parts. Each station (patient assessment, airway, spinal immobilization, and rapid extrication) should be reviewed to include:
1. How to set up each station
2. What equipment and personnel are needed
3. Objectives of the station
4. Helpful hints

Final Assessment Stations

Each station (Final Assessment Stations I, II, and III) should be reviewed to include:
1. How to set up each station
2. What equipment and personnel are needed
3. Objectives of the station
4. Participant performance criteria
5. Helpful hints

Written Examination Overview

During this section, the written evaluation should be reviewed by all participants. Each question should be discussed as directed by participants. All instructor/coordinator candidates should be able to identify the educational objective for each question. Discussion about using the same evaluation for both pre- and post-program should also be held during this section.

Summary

This section should be used to "tie-up" any loose ends or questions participants may have. Participants should also be reminded at this time that they will complete the PHTLS instructor program after successful monitoring by a PHTLS national faculty member during a PHTLS provider program.

LECTURE OUTLINES
Welcome/Introduction

Slide No.	Lecture Content	Notes
I-1	*Title and Logo*	_____
I-2	FOCUS: **Welcome participants, introduce faculty**	_____
I-3	*Instructor Course Objectives*	_____
	FOCUS: **Orient participants to what needs to be accomplished**	
	▪ Identify components of the PHTLS Table of Organization	_____
	▪ Identify the members of the PHTLS Executive Council	_____
	▪ Identify the different PHTLS regions	
	▪ Identify the applicable PHTLS Regional and/or State Coordinator	_____

Slide No.	Lecture Content	Notes

I-4

Instructor Course Objectives—cont'd

- Locate the International PHTLS Office address, phone number, fax, and Web site.
- Identify the different PHTLS programs and who may participate.
- Discuss each station, written examination, and successful course completion.
- Discuss the paperwork shuffle.
- Discuss the set-up of each practical skills station.

I-5

Program Schedule

FOCUS: **Review the plan for the day**

The schedule may change to fit the needs and abilities of the audience.

I-6

Title Slide

Administrative overview

I-7

What We Will Cover Here

FOCUS: **Review the list of items**

- PHTLS organizational structure
- PHTLS executive council members
- NAEMT and ACS/COT affiliation
- PHTLS regions
- PHTLS staff directory

I-8

What We Will Cover Here—cont'd

- PHTLS instructor manual
- Pre- and postcourse paperwork
- International PHTLS office and support material

I-9

PHTLS Table of Organization

FOCUS: **Identify the organizational structure of PHTLS and its relationship to ACS/COT and NAEMT**

I-10

PHTLS Executive Council

FOCUS: **Identify the PHTLS leadership**

The course coordinator should distribute copies of the latest PHTLS directory to each course participant. Go over the directory with the participants, naming the chair, vice-chair, medical director, associate medical director, international coordinator, and education coordinator.

Slide No.	Lecture Content	Notes

I-11 *Detailed PHTLS Organizational Chart*
FOCUS: **Identify levels of PHTLS faculty**

- Executive council
- Regional coordinators
- State coordinators
- Affiliate faculty
- Course coordinators
- Instructors and faculty
- Participants

I-12 *NAEMT*
FOCUS: **Describe NAEMT for the participants**

- Founded in 1975
- Professional representative organization
- Liaison to other related organizations
- Educational programs and conferences
- Parent organization of PHTLS
- Societies
- Are you a member?

I-13 *ACS/COT*
FOCUS: **Discuss the relationship of the American College of Surgeons, Committee on Trauma with PHTLS**

- American College of Surgeons, Committee on Trauma
- Advanced Trauma Life Support (ATLS)
- Medical "soundness" of PHTLS
  - Standard of care
- Cooperation with NAEMT
- Chairperson, state/provincial COT
  - Not required at each program

I-14 *Partnership*
FOCUS: **Emphasize partnership of NAEMT and ACS/COT in PHTLS**

I-15 *PHTLS National Faculty*
FOCUS: **Identify members of the PHTLS national faculty**

Members of the PHTLS national faculty include:

- Members of the PHTLS executive council
- Regional Coordinators
- State Coordinators
- Others approved by the executive council

Slide No.	Lecture Content	Notes

I-16

PHTLS National Faculty—cont'd

- Can be appointed by the chairperson
  - PHTLS Affiliate Faculty
  - PHTLS Instructor/Coordinator
  - Recommendation of Regional/State Coordinator
  - One-time or permanent basis

I-17

PHTLS Regional Coordinators

FOCUS: **Discuss the regions and the regional coordinators and their roles**

- United States divided into three regions
- Military and international regions
- Coordinator for each region
- Appointed by PHTLS chairperson
- Oversees state coordinators and activities within their own region

I-18

PHTLS State Coordinator

FOCUS: **Describe the state coordinators and their roles**

- Appointed by the PHTLS chairperson
  - Provides QA/QI for programs conducted within own state
  - Promotion of PHTLS
  - Works with the state COT

I-19

PHTLS Affiliate Faculty

FOCUS: **Describe the affiliate faculty and their roles**

- PHTLS affiliate faculty are appointed by the chairperson or by the regional or state coordinators.
- Their role is to serve as QA/QI locally when needed.

I-20

Local Host Organization

FOCUS: **Identify and describe the role of the host organization**

- Sponsors a PHTLS program
- Local responsibilities

I-21

Course Medical Director

FOCUS: **Identify the course medical director and his or her role**

The course medical director needs to be:

- A physician
- At least an ATLS provider (preferably an ATLS instructor)
- Available during the program (if not on-site, available by phone)

Slide No.	Lecture Content	Notes

I-22

Course Coordinator

FOCUS: **Identify the course coordinator and his or her role**

- Primary local administrative authority
- PHTLS Instructor/Coordinator.

I-23

PHTLS Instructor/Coordinator

FOCUS: **Identify the instructor/coordinator and his or her role**

- Completed both the provider and instructor program
- Be observed by National Faculty (within 1 year of completing the instructor course)
- Valid for a 3-year period
- Maintain provider status and instruct in at least one PHTLS program annually

I-24

Adjunct Faculty

FOCUS: **Identify adjunct faculty and their roles**

- Specialty instructors
  - Physicians
  - Nurses
  - Other ancillary medical personnel
  - Educators
- Practical skill evaluators
  - PHTLS providers (minimum)
  - Must have skills to evaluate
  - Knowledge of equipment

I-25

Available PHTLS Programs

FOCUS: **Title Slide**

I-26

PHTLS Programs

FOCUS: **Identify the types of PHTLS courses**

- Provider
  - Available for advanced, basic, or combined audiences
- Refresher
  - Available to PHTLS and BTLS providers to give the participants current PHTLS provider status
- Instructor
  - To train instructor/coordinator candidates

I-27

Student Surcharges

FOCUS: **Title slide**

Slide No.	Lecture Content	Notes

I-28

Surcharges

FOCUS: **The specific fees that must be collected per student for each course**

These fees must be collected by the course coordinator and forwarded to the International PHTLS office.

- Provider Program: $15 per participant
- Refresher Program: $10 per participant
- Instructor Program: $10 per participant
- Payment upon completion of the program.

I-29

Continuing Education Coordinating Board for Emergency Medical Services (CECBEMS)

FOCUS: **Title slide**

I-30

CECBEMS

FOCUS: **Fees for CECBEMS credit**

If you would like CECBEMS continuing education credits for your PHTLS program, send an additional $15 per course, along with your other fees and rosters to the PHTLS International Office. Check the box on your course invoice requesting CECBEMS credit. CECBEMS awards 16.25 advanced continuing education hours, 17.9 basic provider hours, or 9.9 hours for the refresher.

I-31

International PHTLS Office

FOCUS: **Title slide**

I-32

International PHTLS Office

FOCUS: **Identify the International PHTLS Office and how to contact it**

408 Monroe Street,
Clinton, Mississippi 39056

Phone: 1-800-94-PHTLS
Fax: 601-924-7325
Website: http://naemt.org/phtls/

I-33

PHTLS Support Materials

FOCUS: **Identify the PHTLS support materials and where they can be found**

- Program brochures
- Slides
- Wallet cards
- Certificates of completion
- Written evaluation (master)
- All forms (master)
- Logo items

Slide No.	Lecture Content	Notes

I-34

PHTLS Slides

FOCUS: **Description of the PHTLS slide set and how to get the slides**

- Copyrighted material
- Only to be used in approved PHTLS programs
- Can be purchased for use by a course site
- Loaned from the PHTLS International Office for a program

I-35

Precourse Paperwork

FOCUS: **Identify the paperwork that needs to be done prior to the course**

- Course planning and approval
- Proposed budget
- Submitted to International PHTLS office, Regional/State Coordinator, and State COT (at least 30 days before program)
- International and state numbers assigned
- Letter of approval, assigning affiliate faculty and program numbers

I-36

International Numbering System for PHTLS Programs

FOCUS: **Title slide**

I-37

Numbering System

FOCUS: **Describe the national numbering system**

Three-part numbering system. Example: 98-0000-00

- 98 = Calendar year of the program
- 0000 = Sequential program number beginning at 0001 each year
- 00 = Type of program

I-38

Program Types (Numbering)

FOCUS: **Describe program numbering system**

- 01 = Basic provider
- 02 = Advanced provider
- 03 = Combined provider
- 04 = Basic instructor
- 05 = Advanced instructor
- 06 = Combined instructor

I-39

Program Types (Numbering)—cont'd

- 07 = Basic provider and instructor
- 08 = Advanced provider and instructor
- 09 = Combined provider and instructor
- 10 = Basic refresher
- 11 = Advanced refresher
- 12 = Combined refresher

Slide No.	Lecture Content	Notes

I-40

Course Coordinator Responsibilities

FOCUS: **Title slide**

I-41

Course Coordinator to Participants

FOCUS: **What the course participants should get from the course coordinator and when**

- Letter
  - Acceptance into program
  - Schedule
  - Dress
- Textbook
- First day of class
  - Group assignments
  - Rotation schedule
  - Lecture evaluation forms and registration forms

I-42

Rotation Groups

FOCUS: **Putting together rotation groups for baseline, teaching, and evaluation stations**

- Alternate participants
- Groups of 3 to 4 individuals
- Work with other services/agencies
- Place identified weaker individuals with stronger individuals
- Change off leader roles

I-43

Student Registration Form

FOCUS: **Describe the form and what should be done with it**

- Copied from the master
- Completed at the beginning of the program
- Keep copies at local site

I-44

Lecture Evaluation

FOCUS: **Describe the lecture evaluation form and what to do with it**

- Copied from master
- One for each lecture
- Completed at end of each lecture and picked up
- Show to each individual instructor
- Maintain with class file

I-45

Course Coordinator to Faculty

FOCUS: **What the faculty should receive from the course coordinator**

- Lecture assignments
  - Outlines and slides
- Skill station assignments
  - Outline/objectives

Slide No.	Lecture Content	Notes

- Final assessment assignments
  - Outline/objectives
- Rotation schedule
- Group assignments

I-46   *International Office to Course Coordinator*

FOCUS: **What the course coordinator can expect to receive from the PHTLS International Office**

- Slides (if needed), 21 days prior to the course
- Invoice
- Certificates and wallet cards

I-47   *Postcourse Paperwork*

FOCUS: **Title slide**

I-48   *Paperwork to International Office*

FOCUS: **What you need to send to the International PHTLS Office on completion of your course**

- Student roster
- Faculty roster
- Invoice copy
- Payment for participant surcharge
- Slides
- Include national course number on all correspondence.

I-49   *Paperwork to State Coordinator*

FOCUS: **What you need to send to your state coordinator upon completion of the course**

- Student roster
- Faculty roster
- Student registrations
- Compiled lecture evaluations
- Compiled course evaluations
- Course summary report

I-50   *Paperwork to Course Coordinator*

FOCUS: **What the course coordinator should keep on file**

- Student roster
- Student registrations
- Pre- and posttest answer sheets
- Compiled lecture evaluations
- Compiled course evaluations
- Course summary report
- Copy of invoice
- Copy of payment

Slide No.	Lecture Content	Notes

I-51

Provider Program

FOCUS: **Title slide**

I-52

Who Can Attend?

FOCUS: **Identify who is eligible to participate in the program**

- EMS providers
  - All levels of prehospital care providers
- Others (with emergency background)
  - Nurses
  - Physician assistants
  - Physicians

I-53

Skills Demonstrated or Practiced throughout the Program **Do Not** *Certify Individuals to Perform Skills that Are Outside of Their Normal Scope of Practice.*

FOCUS: **This slide identifies that the course is not a certification and cannot certify individuals to perform skills they are not licensed or certified to do within their license or practice**

I-54

Schedule for Provider Course

FOCUS: **The focus of the next nine slides is to review the course schedule and the appropriate faculty to perform specific functions**

- Flexible scheduling; 16 hours
- Written precourse Evaluation and Baseline Assessment
  - 30 minutes
  - PHTLS instructors
    Underscore the importance of keeping the course moving. There should be no discussion after the baseline scenario. Inform the students that the scenario will be discussed during the course. Baselines "set the mood" of the course. Keep it lighthearted and keep it moving.
  - Score sheets (these are in the instructor manual)
- Course purpose
  - 15 minutes
  - Course coordinator/affiliate faculty should also discuss what happened in baselines (score sheets).

I-55

Schedule for Provider Course—cont'd

- Kinematics of Trauma
  - 50 minutes
  - "Strong" instructor
    Important lecture sets the tone for the rest of the course.
- Break—15 minutes
- Patient Assessment
  - 50 minutes
  - A B C D E type of person

Slide No.	Lecture Content	Notes

I-56

Schedule for Provider Course—cont'd
- Airway Management
  - 30 minutes
  - Know local area skills
  - Oxygen, oxygen, oxygen, and oxygen
- Lunch—45 minutes
- Shock and Fluid Replacement
  - 45 minutes
  - This is one of the lectures with a fair amount of "advanced" content. Be prepared to cater the lecture to your audience.

I-57

Schedule for Provider Course—cont'd
- Spinal Trauma
  - 30 minutes
  - "Skills" person not needed yet
- Assessment demonstration
  - 15 minutes
  - Video
  - "Live"

It's a good idea to demonstrate the skills for your audience so they get an opportunity to see the "faculty" perform the skills the way you want to see the students perform them. You may want to consider making a video with your faculty to use here.

I-58

Schedule for Provider Course—cont'd
- Practical Skills Station
  - Assessment I
  - Airway Management
  - Spinal Immobilization
  - Rapid Extrication
  - 45-minute rotations
  - Joint Overviews
  - Small "hands on" groups

I-59

Schedule for Provider Course—cont'd
- Considerations in the Elderly and Pediatric Patient
  - 30 minutes
  - Point out the differences in the way elderly and pediatric patients respond to trauma as well as the differences in the approach to assessment in these patients.
- Thoracic Trauma
  - 30 minutes
- Abdominal Trauma and Trauma in Pregnancy
  - 20 minutes

I-60

Schedule for Provider Course—cont'd
- Break
  - 15 minutes

Slide No.	Lecture Content	Notes

- Head Trauma
  - 30 minutes
- Practical Skills Teaching Stations II
  - Assessment II
  - Pediatric Assessment and Immobilization
  - 30-minute rotations

I-61

Schedule for Provider Course—cont'd

- Musculoskeletal Trauma
  - 15 minutes
- Thermal Trauma
  - 30 minutes
  - This lecture covers much ground and can run long if the instructor is not careful.
- Lunch
  - 30 minutes

I-62

Schedule for Provider Course—cont'd

- Essentials in Prehospital care
  - 15 minutes
  - Course Coordinator/Affiliate Faculty
  - Includes course summary
- Final Assessment
  - PHTLS instructors as evaluators
  - Be prepared with alternative scenarios and stations if you need to run extra stations to evaluate individuals as "team leaders" or remediate participants who had problems in a final assessment station.
- Course completion

I-63

Refresher Program

FOCUS: **Title slide**

I-64

Refresher Course

FOCUS: **Review of course schedule and roles of instructors**

- Recommended every 3 years
  - Designed to re-recognize PHTLS providers who took their last course 3 years ago or less. Also for BTLS providers who took their last BTLS course 3 years ago or less and now wish to be recognized as PHTLS providers.
- Instructors who need to maintain their provider status may also use the refresher course to keep their status current.
- This is an 8-hour course, but it can run long if you are not careful. The lectures are lengthy and cover a lot of material quickly. If you have not run a refresher, you should try to get an experienced individual to help you on your first one. Be prepared for some rusty skills during the final evaluations as this course does not have teaching stations.

Slide No.	Lecture Content	Notes

I-65

Schedule for Refresher Course

FOCUS: **Review Refresher Program schedule**

The schedule is flexible but the following is the most typical and most successful template.

- Introduction and Welcome
  - 15 minutes
- Course Purpose
  - 15 minutes
- Instructed by Course Coordinator/Affiliate Faculty

I-66

Schedule for Refresher Course—cont'd

- Managing the Multisystem Trauma Patient–Part I
  - 60 minutes
  - This section is long but there is a great deal of material to cover in the allotted period of time. This lecturer needs to be experienced and comfortable with the entire text.
- Break
  - 15 minutes
- Managing the Multisystem Trauma Patient—Part II
  - 60 minutes
- Break
  - 15 minutes

I-67

Schedule for Refresher Course—cont'd

- Special Considerations in the Elderly and Pediatric Patient
  - 30 minutes
  - This lecture combines the information from both the elderly and pediatric chapters in the textbook. The lecturer needs to be comfortable with both ends of the age dependent considerations spectrum.
- Lunch
  - 60 minutes
- Megatrends in Trauma—What's New, What's Changed, What's Controversial
  - 60 minutes
  - "Strong" person
  - What's new? What's changed? What's controversial? This lecture requires an extremely strong and confident speaker who will be able to present this material, handle controversial topics, and field enthusiastic questions and comments.

I-68

Schedule for Refresher Course—cont'd

- Skill Stations and Written Examination
  - Patient Assessment A and B
  - Airway: Basic and Advanced
  - Spinal Skills A and B
  - Written examination
  - 3 hours
- Course completion

Slide No.	Lecture Content	Notes

I-69

Instructor Program
FOCUS: **Title slide**

I-70

Instructor Program
FOCUS: **Review of eligible participants and schedule**

- 8-hour program
- Who can attend? Anyone with current provider status and a letter of recommendation from his or her course coordinator or national faculty.
- When am I a "real instructor?" Once the candidate has successfully completed the instructor course, he or she will have to be monitored by a national faculty representative while instructing a Provider Program in order to become recognized as an instructor.

I-71

Schedule for Instructor Program
FOCUS: **Review Instructor Program schedule**

- Welcome, Registration, and Introductions
  - 15 minutes
- Administrative Overview
  - 90 minutes
  - Consider a break of 15 minutes about halfway through this lecture.
- Break
  - 15 minutes

I-72

Schedule for Instructor Program—cont'd

- Teaching Techniques
  - 60 minutes
  - This lecture may be done by an "educator." The idea is to learn how to teach. A "PHTLS" person is not necessarily needed.
- Lunch
  - 60 minutes
- Teaching Stations Overview
  - 150 minutes
  - Make sure there is time for the candidates to show how they would present the skills stations.

I-73

Schedule for Instructor Program—cont'd

- Break
  - 15 minutes
- Final Assessment Stations Overview
  - 60 minutes
  - Review each of the stations and give the candidates opportunity to demonstrate their comfort level with running these stations.

Slide No.	Lecture Content	Notes

I-74   *Schedule for Instructor Program—cont'd*
- Written Evaluation Overview
  - 30 minutes
  - Go over each question and make sure the candidates can explain the reasoning behind the answers for each of the questions in the final evaluation.
- Summary
  - 15 minutes

I-75   *PHTLS Program Software*
FOCUS: **Title slide**

I-76   *PHTLS Program Software*
FOCUS: **Identify the PHTLS program software, its uses, and how to get it**
- PHTLS "Management System"
- Automated creation of:
  - All course forms
  - Course documentation
- Database
  - Participants
  - Faculty

I-77   *PHTLS Program Software—cont'd*
- IBM
  - 80386/25 CPU
  - DOS 5.0
  - Windows 3.1
  - 8MB RAM
  - 550K Lower Memory
  - 10MB hard drive space
  - Inkjet printer
  - Laser printer

I-78   *PHTLS Program Software—cont'd*
- Macintosh
  - 68020 CPU
  - System 7.x
  - 8MB RAM
  - 10MB hard drive space
  - Inkjet printer
  - Laser printer

Slide No.	Lecture Content	Notes

I-79

PHTLS Program Software—cont'd
- Different level programs for state/regional coordinators
- Must be approved by International Office to purchase

I-80

Teaching Techniques
FOCUS: **Title slide**

I-81

Objectives
FOCUS: **Review objectives**
- The participant will be able to:
  - List activities to enhance PHTLS teaching and learning
  - Apply the art and science of adult learning to PHTLS
  - Use advanced educational taxonomies during PHTLS instruction

I-82

Teaching
FOCUS: **Acknowledge all have own style**
- Teaching "how to teach" is a challenging task.
- We each develop a unique teaching style that is often influenced by those teachers whose styles we have admired.
- Our teaching styles are usually a result of one of our teachers who we admired—not education.
- Good teachers learn to combine educational theory with personal teaching styles and methods.

I-83

Teaching Defined
- A planned experience that brings about a change in behavior (learning)

I-84

Change
FOCUS: **Identifying change**
- Concept of change may be applied when we know:
  - The ideal performance standards
  - The actual performance—observing baselines, skill stations, the pretest
  - The gap between ideal standards and actual standards of performance—talk with the instructors, visit with the students, observe the stations, find the gaps so change can occur

I-85

Goal of Teaching
FOCUS: **Instruction should fill knowledge gap**
The goal of teaching is to design and deliver instruction that will guide the actual performance to the ideal—fill the gap.

Slide No.	Lecture Content	Notes

I-86

PHTLS Teaching Skills

FOCUS: **The skills needed for teaching**

- Lecture
- Questioning
- Discussion
- Skills stations
- Scenario presentations

I-87

The Lecture

FOCUS: **Advantages and disadvantages**

- Advantage
  - Consistent, efficient delivery of information
- Disadvantage
  - Material is not well retained

I-88

The Lecturer

FOCUS: **Maintain interest while imparting knowledge**

- Educator must be dynamic to maintain students' interest.
- A vast amount of knowledge does not make a good lecturer.
- Lecturing/entertainment skills must complement the teacher's presentation of information.

I-89

Lecture Keys

FOCUS: **Lecture must accommodate needs of audience**

- Know your audience (i.e., level of training, where they work).
- Know where change needs to occur. (Watch baselines, review students' written exams for trends, talk to the students.)
- Direct your lecture to meet the students' needs or to fill the gap.
- Stay focused and on topic—you have limited time.
- Use repetitions

I-90

Lecture Preparation

FOCUS: **Preparing for lecture**

- Read the chapter.
- Review the outline.
- Review the slides.
- Review outline and slides together.
- Practice, practice, practice
- Avoid practicing failure. (If you are going through your lecture and make a mistake or mess up, stop, go back, and correct yourself so your brain remembers the lecture the way you want to deliver it.)

Slide No.	Lecture Content	Notes

I-91

Preparing YOUR Lecture

FOCUS: **Using PHTLS materials effectively**

- Take the outline and make it your own.
- Be aware of how the slides complement your lecture. Slides have focus points in the outline to remind you why it is there.
- Be prepared, so you look prepared.

I-92

Successful Lecture

FOCUS: **Keys to successful lecture**

- Keep points to a minimum.
- Summarize often, remembering that 80% of the information you provide will be forgotten within 8 weeks.
- You can't teach skills.
- It is OK to *not* know it all.

I-93

Consider Mental Processing

FOCUS: **People process information differently at different times**

Everyone processes with both parts of their brain. Some will rely on the left and others on the right depending on the hat they are wearing.

- Left
  - Verbal—words
  - Symbols—words can be symbols for things, some icons
  - Temporal—time-oriented
  - Rational—cause and effect
  - Logical—orderly flow
  - Linear—one way through, outline
  - Concepts—The left side of the brain deals best with concepts.
- Right
  - Nonverbal—pictures, drawings, handling the object
  - Concrete—realistic, words will be taken literally
  - Nontemporal—not time conscious at all
  - Nonrational
  - Intuitive—come to the same conclusion, but cannot tell you how they got there
  - Wholistic—see the problem as a whole but cannot break down into individual steps, scattered
  - Experience—the right side of the brain deals best with experiences.

I-94

Left Brain Tools

FOCUS: **Tools and examples for left brain processing**

- Outline—Give the left brain students an outline; the right brain students will probably ignore it totally.
- Principle—Tell them the guidelines, goals, and limitations.

- Eleven relationships—When designing lectures for the left brain students, these activities may help. However, you cannot use them all.
  - Sameness—how something is like another thing (i.e., The heart is like a pump.)
  - Oppositeness—how something is different from another (i.e., increased ICP vs. shock vital signs)
  - Difference of degree (i.e., burns)
  - Things of the same class (i.e., injuries that cause a decrease in breath sounds)
  - Classification order (i.e., blood vessel size and order, arteries, arterioles, capillaries)
  - A whole and its parts (i.e., the spine broken down into parts—vertebrae, spinal fluid, cord)
  - Steps in a procedure (i.e., description of the up-and-over pathway)
  - Function—How something works (i.e., the heart)
  - Qualities of a thing (i.e., description of Cushing's triad)
  - Cause and effect (i.e., kinematics impacts)
  - A symbol and what it represents (i.e., clock—time ticking away, Golden Hour, Platinum 10 Minutes)

I-95

Right Brain Tools

FOCUS: **Tools and examples for right brain processing**

- Map (i.e., a drawing depicting the direction to take)
- Example (i.e., showing a frontal impact, a lacerated liver)
- Parable—telling a story to make a point (i.e., the Bible, Aesop's Fables)
- Metaphor—a figure of speech in which a word or phrase depicting an object is used in place of another to suggest a likeness [i.e., Paper-bag syndrome occurs in the lungs (use of the word paper bag instead of pneumo); a ship plows the sea (correlation to a tractor plowing); "a stitch in time saves nine" (correlated to the idea of fixing things when you first find them so that they will not be broken the next time you need them)
- Concrete words (i.e., shock—using the words cold, wet, and slimy to describe skin rather than the words cool and diaphoretic)
- Image—visually taking students through an activity (i.e., tour of the heart, diagram of intubation.) Very strong Olympic athletes visualize their sports. Watch them prepare. Their bodies even respond.
- Mime—acting something out (i.e., impacts, injury patterns)

I-96

Lecture Organization

FOCUS: **Organizing a polished lecture**

- Attention grabber—can be a joke (tell good jokes and relate them to content), slide, or activity
  - For example, for abdominal trauma, place some objects in small paper bags and staple bags shut. Then throw a few of

Slide No.	Lecture Content	Notes

the bags out to the class. Have them try to guess what is in the bag. Then go to the abdominal trauma lecture and associate the index of suspicion to guessing what is in the bag.

- Introduction
  - Outline and/or map of where lecture is to go
  - Ground rules (for questions, discussion)
  - Motivation—tie in your attention getter
- Body
  - Do not say too much.
  - Clear transitions—slides help with transitions
- Summary
  - Review main points.
  - Relate back to your introduction.
  - Ask for questions. If there are no questions, then go to the closer.
- Curtain closer
  - A slide (PHTLS has a key point slide to end each lecture) or an activity (Open the bags and see what is inside.)
  - Thank the participants and leave the lectern.
  - Do not ask for more questions.
- This format will make you look professional and polished

I-97

Lecture Techniques

FOCUS: **Lecture presentation techniques**

- Relax
- Involve the students. PHTLS has questions built into the slides.
- Be comfortable with not knowing everything.
- Vary the pace and pitch of your delivery. Do not read to the audience and do not be monotonous.
- Maintain eye contact. Find friendly eyes and look around the room.
- Avoid distractions—if you tend to play with change in your pocket, take it out. If you use words repetitively, make a list of options to remind you or help you. If you have a friend in the audience, have that person let you know when you are repeating the same word over and over again—you will never hear it.

I-98

Lecture Props

FOCUS: **Discussion of lecture props**

- Lighting
  - Keep some type of light on in the room if you have to darken it completely to show slides. Bring in a home or office lamp in order to read your notes.
  - Make sure this light allows the room to be dark enough for viewing slides.
- Microphones
  - Be careful of feedback
  - Change the microphone type to match your style
  - This requires preplanning

Slide No.	Lecture Content	Notes

- Equipment
  - Make sure all equipment is present and in working order before the lecture.
- Notes
  - Your handwriting should be large enough to read from the lectern without holding the notes closer.
  - Organize your notes with a numbering or lettering system so if they get dropped or mixed up, you can put them back in order quickly.
- Audiovisual materials
  - Make sure the AV equipment works.
  - Make sure to load slides correctly. (It is a good idea to project a slide while loading to be certain they are not all upside down or backwards.)
  - Do not use slides with too much information.

I-99

Questions

FOCUS: **How questions can be used in lecture**

- Tie in previous material
- Determine knowledge and experience
- Assist in presenting material
- Stress key points
- Motivate group and maintain attention

I-100

Question Types

FOCUS: **Discuss the question types and uses**

- Recall—ability to provide memorized facts. A few questions like this are OK, especially for early involvement or in general to create a safe environment.
- Application—requires correlating a concept to an experience or an experience to a concept
- Problem solving—provides students with a problem or scenario and asks for solutions. These questions are good for discussion, but watch the time and stay focused.

I-101

Successful Questioning

FOCUS: **Successful questioning techniques**

- Ask specific questions with specific answers. Even with problem-solving questions you can give a scenario and then guide students back to dealing with just the airway problem and issues, for example.
- Use open-ended questions.
- Give the student time to answer (8 seconds). It takes that long to process an answer, especially when problem solving. This can seem like a long time to wait if you are nervous.
- Do not allow one student to dominate.
- Reinforce positive answers.

Slide No.	Lecture Content	Notes

I-102

Questions Generate Discussion

FOCUS: **Using and controlling discussion questions**

- Direct discussions by:
  - Establishing expectations, i.e, set a time limit for each question
  - Controlling participation—call on students if class is out of control or not participating
  - Controlling content—stay on topic
  - Being time conscious—enforce time limits even if just your mental limit
  - Maintaining a positive learning environment
  - Choosing the appropriate teaching strategies—use the appropriate type of questioning for the topic and group

I-103

Discussion: Challenges

FOCUS: **Managing challenging question activities**

- Students give wrong answers.
  - Redirect and let them answer again.
  - Give them a hint.
  - If partially correct, reinforce the correct part and then go to the next student for the remainder.
  - Keep environment positive.
- One student dominates.
  - Call on students by name for answers.

I-104

Teaching Summary

FOCUS: **Summarize teaching portion of lecture**

- Effective teaching using a lecture format depends on your ability to:
  - Set goals
  - Plan
  - Prepare
  - Question and discuss effectively

I-105

PHTLS and Taxonomies

FOCUS: **Domains of learning**

- Cognitive
- Psychomotor
- Affective

I-106

Taxonomies

- Bloom's Cognitive Domain
  - Knowledge—items of factual information (i.e., define paradoxical movement)
  - Comprehension—understanding; obtaining meaning from communication (What does PHTLS say about standing immobilization?)

Slide No.	Lecture Content	Notes

– Application—using information, principles, and the like to solve problems. (Given the material you have received on mechanism of injury, what type of injuries should you suspect looking at the damage during this MVA?)

– Analysis—arriving at an understanding by looking at individual parts. (During baselines, what was the implication of the following signs and symptoms: difficulty breathing, had a rapid respiratory rate, was using accessory muscles?)

– Synthesis—arriving at an understanding by looking at the larger structure, by combining individual elements. (What were this patient's problems?)

– Evaluation—arriving at a value judgment. (Given what you've received in this course, what did you perform well in this scenario?)

▪ A student can operate at the higher levels if guided by the instructor—questioning is a valuable tool

I-107 *Taxonomies*

▪ Bloom's Psychomotor Domain
– Imitation—performing skill like it is demonstrated (i.e., helmet removal)
– Manipulation—changing the skill to do it one's own way, developing a style (i.e., rapid extrication)
– Precision—practice skill until it is second nature (i.e., airway skills)
– Articulation—fits the individual skill into other skills (i.e., combine assessment with airway with rapid extrication—baselines)
– Naturalization—knows when, where skill can be done (i.e., refinement of the skill combinations from baselines to finals)

▪ In order to operate at the higher levels, the student needs planned practice sessions

I-108 *Taxonomies*

▪ Bloom's Affective Domain
– Receiving—willingness to receive stimuli or information (i.e., student chooses to take PHTLS class)
– Responding—responding to information, going beyond reception (i.e., student questions PHTLS material)
– Valuing responding in a way that indicates information has a worth (i.e., student changes behavior in response to PHTLS information or scenarios on next scenario or station)
– Organization—responding in a way that indicates values are in a system and prioritizes the values (i.e., during a scenario, team emphasizes airway as a priority when subtle signs and symptoms of airway difficulty are presented)
– Characterization—internalizes the information into a system to become a philosophy (i.e., student consistently listens to lung sounds as part of the primary when not done before)

Slide No.	Lecture Content	Notes

- It is more difficult to evaluate when you can't follow up with a group—PHTLS creates higher level functioning in the affective domain.

I-109   *Definition of Learning*

FOCUS: **What learning is**

- Learning: a relatively permanent change in behavior which comes about as a result of a planned experience.
- Two key points
  - **Change in behavior**—may be a knowledge, attitude, or skill change
  - **Planned experience**—we must plan when we teach to increase the possibility for change.

I-110   *Adult Learners*

FOCUS: **Characteristics of adult learners**

- Motivation
  - Most adults are self-motivated, but a nudge does not hurt (i.e., baselines or the written pretest).
- Meaningful
  - Information must be meaningful. Make scenarios meaningful, tell war stories, know your audience.
- Active involvement
  - Keep students involved. You need to facilitate learning. Learning is a cooperative venture.
- Self-directed
  - Students need to have input on what and how they learn. Questioning and discussion during lectures and the ability for students to provide input during skill and final stations are all important.

I-111   *Learning*

FOCUS: **Review laws of learning**

- Law of Effects
  - Provide the learner with the needed information and learning will take place.

PHTLS does this in a multitude of ways with lectures, slides, skills, simulations, text, faculty, and other students. Be available, be prepared, and have everything available to the student for stations.

- Law of Readiness
  - If a participant is ready for connections to occur, learning is enhanced.
  - Lectures in PHTLS prepare a student for the connections to occur—war stories may help.
  - Associated stations should follow lectures to enhance the possibility for connections.
  - When possible listen to the lecture if you are overseeing the corresponding station.

- Law of Exercise
  - Repetition of meaningful connections results in learning.
  - PHTLS does this well by building on previous lectures.
  - Skill and final stations reinforce lecture material by helping to make it meaningful.

I-112   *Learning—Summary*

FOCUS: **Review**

- We learn best when we direct our own learning.
- We learn best in context.
- We learn from each other.
- We continuously create knowledge.
- We learn in a learning environment

I-113   *Skills*

FOCUS: **Applying Gardner's levels to PHTLS**

- Gardner's Level of Skills Development
  - Public to private
    - The student needs to manipulate or handle the objects (i.e., airway).
    - The student may do a lot of verbalizing when initially learning steps or when applying information in a new setting.
  - Goal is to get students to apply skills with:
    - Poise—ability to complete skill under great pressure
    - Control—ability to complete skill in a very exacting or fine-tuned manner
    - Timing—ability to know exactly when to complete the skill so that everything will flow
    - Craft—knowing how to apply the skill in a multitude of situations and to be able to adapt and problem solve

I-114   *Skill Station Set-up*

FOCUS: **Preparing for practice skills**

Set-up

- Know the station goal.
- Equipment present and in working order
- Have enough equipment
- Patient present and coached
- Safety concerns—watch skills so no one is injured, patient or students

I-115   *Running the Skill Station*

Delivery

- Orient students—remind them which station they are at. Do not let them get out of order or the whole class will then get mixed up.
- Demonstrate the skill.
- Instructor talk through
  - Demonstration and talk through can be done at the same time.

Slide No.	Lecture Content	Notes

- Student talk through
- Practice with positive reinforcement
- Practice, practice, practice

I-116   *Skill Station Keys*

- Keys
  - We remember it as we see it, so do it right the first time.
  - Stick to topic.
  - Build in time for questions.
  - Decide skill performance ahead of time.
  - Make sure all stations are presented the same.

I-117   *Scenario—Final Station*

FOCUS: **How to prepare the final station**

- Know the station flow.
- Equipment present and in working order
- Enough equipment to do the job for all groups
- Be sure patient is present and moulage is appropriate. Coach patient to respond to your cues.
- Know the critical errors.
- Safety concerns

I-118   *Final Stations Delivery*

- Know the scenario so that you can give immediate feedback to the team.
- Stay where you can see.
- If students don't do it, it's not done.
- Real time is key.
- Keep the scenario the same for all groups.
- Have extra equipment available so you can see what other choices the teams might have made.

I-119   *Final Station*

FOCUS: **Keys to the final station**

Keys

- Doing the scenario in real time
- Let the patient give as much of the information as possible—patient makes the station
- Require skills to be done.
- Force the students to prioritize skills, choose equipment, troubleshoot, delegate, and communicate.

I-120   *Know What Is Passing*

FOCUS: **Be prepared to give positive and negative evaluations**

- Encourage students to evaluate themselves.
- Give feedback according to time.

Slide No.	Lecture Content	Notes

- Give feedback based on critical error criteria, both positive and areas for improvement.
- Do not be afraid to retest someone.
- If more than 50% students pass . . .

I-121

Teaching Summary

- Prepared teachers who enjoy their work, produce prepared students who enjoy their work.
- Have Fun!

I-122

Questions

FOCUS: **Answer questions from participants**

SECTION IV

IV

Refresher Program

PART 1:
Administration

COURSE INTRODUCTION

Authorization/sponsorship: The Prehospital Trauma Life Support (PHTLS) refresher course is a continuing education course by the National Association of Emergency Medical Technicians (NAEMT) in cooperation with the Committee on Trauma (COT) of the American College of Surgeons (ACS).

Course purpose: To review and extend the content of the PHTLS provider course and to reaffirm its knowledge base and key skills.

Who can conduct a course: Any host with proper facilities and faculty as approved by the state PHTLS coordinator in consultation with the state COT chairperson.

Length/time: This 8-hour course may be presented in a 1-day course, 2 half-days, or 3-evening options as possible alternatives.

Term of recognition: All PHTLS certificates are issued for a 3-year recognition period.

Surcharge/costs: A surcharge of $10 for each participant is paid to NAEMT by the host organization, which is responsible for all course costs. The student tuition fee charged is at the discretion of the host.

Level of course: The course is designed for both basic and advanced providers, eliminating the need to run separate courses for each.

Prerequisite requirements for participants: Successful completion of any PHTLS or BTLS provider course (any level) *and* current state or county certification/licensure as an EMT (any level) or currently a nurse, physician assistant, or physician. For military and international courses, an acceptable equivalent of a current certification/licensure is an option.

GOALS AND OBJECTIVES

1. To **review** the key content of the PHTLS course

2. To **expand** the participant's knowledge and understanding of the special considerations in assessment and management of the pediatric and the elderly trauma victim

3. To **revise** and update information previously taught as needed and make the participant aware of current changes and controversies including an understanding of the basis of these changes

4. To **identify:**
   a) Which changes in the state-of-the-art technology result in present changes in the recommended prehospital trauma care
   b) Which changes are controversial and discretionary and may result in differing practices from place to place
   c) Which changes should be recognized as areas of present study and reevaluation but as yet are not resolved by enough data to validate change

5. To **reinforce** that any change in participant's patient care practices requires approval by the local medical authority or the service's medical director

6. To **reaffirm** that the participant has the content knowledge and ability to perform the key skills identified in PHTLS as the recommended prehospital trauma care standard

It is also a goal of the PHTLS refresher course to meet the objectives listed above in an efficient, cost-effective, and time-effective way for participants and those hosting the course. It should also be a dynamic learning experience that avoids unnecessary redundancy in presentation or in achieving the knowledge and skill affirmation. In keeping with this, the refresher course is an 8-hour course and is designed to include basic and advanced personnel, eliminating the need for separate courses for each.

STUDENT QUALIFICATIONS AND SELECTION

This course is designed to provide specific knowledge and skills in prehospital trauma care to the experienced emergency medical technician (basic, intermediate, or paramedic) who has successfully completed a PHTLS or BTLS provider course within the past 3 years. Prehospital personnel selected for the PHTLS refresher course shall be currently state-certified, licensed or certified by the National Registry as emergency medical technician (basic, intermediate, or paramedic). Military personnel who do not necessarily meet these state or national requirements must contact the military coordinator for prior approval.

Participants in international courses shall hold the same provider status as was previously deemed an EMT equivalent for their initial course or shall be required to submit their status in writing to the PHTLS international coordinator and country/territory coordinator for ruling on their equivalency status prior to the course.

All participants are required to furnish a photocopy of their PHTLS provider completion certificate (or card) or BTLS provider completion certificate (or card) *and* a photocopy of their current state or county certification or license to the course coordinator prior to (or at registration for) the refresher course.

If proof of successful completion has been lost or destroyed, a participant should write to the PHTLS International Office (or BTLS National Office) well in advance of the course to ensure receipt of a duplicate by the course date.

COURSE ADMINISTRATION

Class Size

The number of participants for proper learning in any course is dependent on many factors: faculty, course design, facilities, equipment, staffing, and administration.

The PHTLS refresher course contains lectures, a written examination, and skill stations. The number of participants who can be involved in a lecture or take the written examination is limited solely by the size and nature of the facility used for each class. Size does not affect the time required for these courses. The efficiency of, and time required for, each participant to be able to go through each skill station is, however, directly affected by the class size, and therefore it becomes the key limiting factor. In order to run the course within the time frames outlined and avoid participants being unduly delayed for lack of an available open station, the following guidelines should be considered:

> 20 to 24 participants—one of each skill station
> 25 to 48 participants—two of each skill station
> (and an additional staff person to direct participants)
> 49 to 68 participants—three of each skill station
> (and an additional staff person to direct participants)

In cases where personnel or equipment limitations represent a problem, for courses with 25 to 32 participants, or 49 to 64 participants, the following options are possible:

> 25 to 32 participants—one of each station
> (add 30 minutes to expected time)
> 49 to 64 participants—two of each station
> (add 30 minutes to expected time)

Standardization

An essential element in the dissemination of this course is the precise and consistent duplication of the national standard materials and content. No deviations in content are permitted. Instructors may elect to remove individual slides from the sets provided for each lecture as long as the schedule, equipment list, materials, or structure of the PHTLS refresher course is approved in advance and in writing by the regional/state coordinator. Such approval should not be presumed. The PHTLS refresher course is designed to be taught in a time frame of 8 hours, excluding time for a lunch period.

Term of Recognition

The term of recognition for PHTLS initial provider courses and for PHTLS refresher courses is 3 years from the date of completion. It is therefore the recommendation of the PHTLS program that prehospital providers take a refresher class no later than 3 years from their original provider course or 3 years from their last refresher course.

Certificates of successful completion and cards issued for initial provider and refresher courses will, in keeping with this policy, indicate the term of recognition by bearing an expiration date reflecting 3 years from the date of course completion. Admission to a refresher course should occur prior to the participants' expiration date.

In cases where an individual has been unable to take a refresher program course, coordinators can admit an individual into a refresher course for up to 6 months beyond his or her expiration date upon receipt of a letter from the service medical director attesting to the individual's active status and so recommending. This does not extend or change the term of recognition for the individual or alter his or her expiration date; it solely reflects an extended period within which the individual will be allowed into a refresher course.

Except as provided for in the preceding parts of this section, any others seeking to reinstate their term of recognition after their expiration date, shall be required to take a full provider course.

Sponsorship Citations

Sponsorship citations follow the same guidelines established by the National Association of Emergency Medical Technicians Prehospital Trauma Life Support Program. For further details please refer to Section V of this manual.

Student Per Capita Surcharge

A per student surcharge of $10 is paid to NAEMT/PHTLS by the host organization as part of the course finances within 30 days of completion of the course. All course fees must be forwarded to PHTLS International Office, 408 Monroe Street, Clinton, Mississippi 39056.

Budgeting

   Adjunct faculty
   Facilities
   Materials and equipment
   NAEMT student surcharge ($10 per student)

Budgeting follows the same recommendations established by the National Association of Emergency Medical Technicians Prehospital Trauma Life Support Program. For further details please refer to Section V of this manual.

PHTLS Promotion Items

All orders for promotion items should be referred to PHTLS International Office, 408 Monroe Street, Clinton, Mississippi 39056.

Written Materials

A master copy of all handout materials related to the refresher course, evaluation forms, skill station, and situational exercise forms and instructions can be found in this manual. The host organization is responsible for either purchasing or duplicating the master copies in appropriate quantities to ensure successful conduct of the course. The PHTLS provider and instructor text may be purchased directly from the publisher, Mosby, Inc.

Slides

Slides for the PHTLS refresher course are copyrighted material and are the property of NAEMT. No reproduction of these slides is permitted in any form. The slides are loaned or purchased to the host organization for use exclusively in the approved PHTLS refresher course. Slides will be sent to the course coordinator well in advance of the course date by the PHTLS International Office. Should the slides not be received by 21 days before the course date, the course coordinator should call the PHTLS International Office. The lecture outlines include a precise description of each slide and indicate its placement in the lecture's sequence. The course coordinator is responsible to collect the slides after the course and to mail them back to the PHTLS International Office within 2 weeks of the course's completion if the slides have been loaned and not purchased.

Written Examinations

Written examinations follow the same guidelines established by the National Association of Emergency Medical Technicians Prehospital Trauma Life Support Program. For further details please refer to Section V of this manual.

Registration Form

Registration forms follow the same guidelines established by the National Association of Emergency Medical Technicians Prehospital Trauma Life Support Program. For further details please refer to Section V of this manual.

Certificates/Wallet Cards

Certificates and wallet cards follow the same guidelines established by the National Association of Emergency Medical Technicians Prehospital Trauma Life Support Program.

Evaluation Form

A Refresher Course Evaluation Form can be found in Section V. This is to be completed by each student and collected by the course coordinator at the end of the course. These evaluation forms should be sent with the course summary report to the state coordinator. These will be summarized and a copy of the summary is forwarded to the state COT chairperson, course co-ordinator, and course medical director.

Summary Report

A Refresher Course Summary Report is completed during the course by the course coordinator and signed by the course coordinator, course medical director, and affiliate faculty. This form summarizes the course in one form and includes the date, location, host, key personnel, faculty, and students' names and addresses. The completed form becomes the permanent NAEMT record of the course. The course coordinator is responsible for having these postcourse materials sent *no later than 10 days* from the course completion date.

Equipment and Supplies

A list of the needed equipment and supplies is required, and variances are not permitted without advanced written approval from the state/regional co-ordinator. The quantities on the list are based upon enrollment.

Facilities

Facilities follow the same recommendations established by the National Association of Emergency Medical Technicians Prehospital Trauma Life Support Program. For further details please refer to Section V of this manual.

Refresher Course Application

The Refresher Application Form and the Proposed Budget and Faculty Form *must* be completed and sent together to the PHTLS state coordinator (or PHTLS regional coordinator in states where no state coordinator has been identified). *These must be received by the state coordinator no later than 90 days in advance of the proposed course date(s).*

If you do not know the PHTLS coordinator for your state, his/her name, address, and phone number can be obtained by calling the International PHTLS Office, in Clinton, Mississippi.

Telephone: (800) 94-PHTLS

FAX: 601-924-7325

Address: PHTLS International Office
408 Monroe Street
Clinton, Mississippi 39056

REFRESHER COURSE SCHEDULE

The PHTLS refresher course is designed to be a high-intensity learning and affirmation experience. The best dynamics for this are achieved in a single day focused on trauma. The continuous and uninterrupted developmental interaction between faculty and participants greatly enhances the group dynamics, learning, and impact of the course on the participant's performance. The 1-day format is the preferred and recommended choice.

Prehospital Trauma Life Support

In cases where local resources (or factors surrounding participant's work schedules) will not allow for the 1-day format, two other schedules are provided:
- a 2 half-day schedule
- a 3-evening schedule

Classically, evening continuing education sessions have been limited to 3 hours, requiring 3 evenings to complete the course. Where evenings can be scheduled for 4-1/2 hours, the 2 half-day schedule can be used. In either of these options, the course should usually be completed within 2 weeks. It is required that, in any format, a course must be completed within 30 days from its starting date.

No change in course content, scope, or sequence is allowed.

1-Day Schedule

8:00–8:15 am	Introduction and Welcome	(15 min)
8:15–8:30 am	Refresher Course Purpose	(15 min)
8:30–9:30 am	Managing the Multisystem Trauma Patient—Part I	(1 hr)
8:30–9:45 am	Break	(15 min)
9:45–10:45 am	Managing the Multisystem Trauma Patient—Part II	(1 hr)
10:45–11:00 am	Break	(15 min)
11:00–11:30 am	Special Considerations in Elderly and Pediatric Patients	(30 min)
11:30–12:30 pm	Lunch	(1 hr)
12:30–1:30 pm	Megatrends in Trauma	(1 hr)
1:30–1:35 pm	Read Instructions for Skill Stations and Written Test	(5 min)
1:35–2:35 pm	Written Test	(1 hr)
2:00*–5:00 pm	Skill Station Rotations	(3 hr)
	1. Patient Assessment "A""	
	2. Patient Assessment "B"	
	3. Airway and Ventilation	
	4. Advanced Airway and Thoracentesis Advanced personnel only	
	5. Spine Skills "A" Logrolls and Standing Longboard	
	6. Spine Skills "B" Rapid Extrication	
5:00–End	Completion—Give out results/certificates	
5:00–5:30 pm	Individual remediation, as needed	

*Since some participants will complete the written test in 30 minutes or less, skill stations should be ready to start at this time.

Alternate, 2 Half-Day Schedule

1st Half Day

8:00–8:15 am	12:30–12:45 pm	Introduction and Welcome	(15 min)
8:15–8:30 am	12:45–1:00 pm	Refresher Course Purpose	(15 min)
8:30–9:30 am	1:00–2:00 pm	Managing the Multisystem Trauma Patient—Part I	(1 hr)
9:30–10:00 am	2:00–2:30 pm	Break	(30 min)
10:00–11:00 am	2:30–3:30 pm	Managing the Multisystem Trauma Patient—Part II	(1 hr)
11:00–11:30 am	3:30–4:00 pm	Break	(30 min)
11:30–12:00 noon	4:00–4:30 pm	Special Considerations in Elderly and Pediatric Patients	(30 min)

2nd Half Day

8:00–9:00 am	12:30–1:30 pm	Megatrends in Trauma	(1 hr)
9:00–9:05 am	1:30–1:35 pm	Read Instructions for Skill Stations and Written Test	(5 min)
9:05–10:05 am	1:35–2:35 pm	Written Test	(1 hr)
9:30*–12:00 noon	2:00*–4:30 pm	Skill Station Rotations	(2.5 hr)
		1. Patient Assessment "A"	
		2. Patient Assessment "B"	
		3. Airway and Ventilation	
		4. Advanced Airway and Thoracentesis	
		5. Spine Skills "A" Logrolls and Standing Longboard	
		6. Spine Skills "B" Rapid Extrication	
12:00–End	4:30–End	Completion—Give out results/ certificates	
12:00–1:00 pm	4:30–5:30 pm	Individual remediation, as needed	

*Since some participants will complete the written test in 30 minutes or less, skill stations should be ready to start at this time.

Alternate, 3-Evening Schedule

1st Evening

7:00*–7:15 pm	Introductions and Welcome	(15 min)
7:15–7:30 pm	Refresher Course Purpose	(15 min)
7:30–8:30 pm	Managing the Multisystem Trauma Patient—Part I	(1 hr)
8:30–8:45 pm	Break	(15 min)
8:45–9:45 pm	Managing the Multisystem Trauma Patient—Part II	(1 hr)

2nd Evening

7:00*–7:30 pm	Special Considerations in Elderly and Pediatric Patients	(30 min)
7:30–7:45 pm	Break	(15 min)
7:45–8:45 pm	Megatrends in Trauma	(1 hr)
8:45–9:00 pm	Break	(15 min)
9:00–10:00 pm	Written Test	(1 hr)

3rd Evening

7:00–7:05 pm	Read Instructions for Skill Stations and Written Test	(5 min)
7:05–9:35 pm	Skill Station Rotations	(2.5 hr)
	1. Patient Assessment "A"	
	2. Patient Assessment "B"	
	3. Airway and Ventilation	
	4. Advanced Airway and Thoracentesis (ALS only)	
	5. Spine Skills "A"	
	Logrolls and Standing Longboard	
	6. Spine Skills "B"	
	Rapid Extrication	
9:35–End	Completion—Give out results/certificates	
9:35–10:05 pm	Individual remediation, as needed	

*The evening schedule can start at 5:50 pm, 6:00 pm, 6:30 pm, etc., adjusting times accordingly; 7:00 pm is used simply as an example.

REFRESHER COURSE CONTENTS

The detailed contents of each lecture (including slides) and of each of the skill stations in this course are presented at the end of this section. An overview of the contents of each is provided here as an aid to the reader.

Lecture 1—Refresher Course Purpose   (15 min)

Immediately following the welcome and introductions, the PHTLS affiliate faculty for the course briefly introduces the "purpose" of the course: to review in a short, precise form the Management of the Multisystem Trauma Patient presented in the provider course; to extend the participants' knowledge of Special Considerations in Pediatric Trauma and Trauma of the Elderly; to highlight recent changes in trauma care (or changes from earlier courses) and to identify areas that remain controversial; to affirm and improve participants' ability to perform key skills in hands-on skill stations and to gauge their knowledge with a course-end test.

Lecture 2—Managing the Multisystem
Trauma Patient—Part I (1 hr)

In a precise review, this lecture highlights the following: an overview of trauma and its national impact; the kinematics of blunt and penetrating trauma; patient assessment; airway and ventilation management and oxygenation; circulation and shock; PASG; and fluid resuscitation.

Lecture 3—Managing the Multisystem
Trauma Patient—Part II (1 hr)

This lecture reviews and highlights key considerations in the following: thoracic trauma, abdominal trauma, head trauma, spine trauma, extremity trauma, and burn trauma. It closes with a summary of the management of patients with multisystem trauma and simple, isolated trauma.

Lecture 4—Special Considerations in Elderly
and Pediatric Patients (30 min)

This lecture starts by establishing that critically injured children and older adults require the same priorities of assessment and resuscitation as younger adults. The lecture continues with the following: the respiratory and circulatory compensation in children (emphasizing the ability to compensate for a longer period of time and the resultant sudden decompensation that occurs); the need to treat respiratory distress and signs of early shock aggressively before profound shock or exhaustion and respiratory arrest occurs; thoracic differences (such that even a single rib fracture must be assumed to have a life-threatening injury associated with it); extremity injury, growth plate considerations, and the serious potential implication on growth of what in older patients would be considered minor injuries; and required differences in method and equipment for spinal immobilization and other areas.

After defining which patients must be considered elderly, this lecture discusses the following: the normal pathophysiology of aging; its effect on the healthy elderly patient's ability to withstand trauma; common significant medical problems and their ongoing chronic effects on the body; effects of medications on the assessment findings and on the patient's ability to compensate; awareness of and need for inclusion of age, general physical condition, medical history and problems, and medications in assessment and management of elderly trauma victims. Finally, this lecture discusses the approach to elderly patients and their mental status.

Lecture 5—Megatrends in Trauma (1 hr)

This lecture is designed to make participants aware of changes in current trauma care, identifying changes from earlier teachings and practices. It includes the following, with clear distinction: commonly accepted changes in standards of care; changes which result in differing conclusions and local practices; and controversies that remain, requiring more scientific study. The contents of this lecture are reviewed frequently and will be updated as studies are done and the literature changes. The lecture presently includes such topics as PASG and fluid resuscitation, advanced airway adjuncts, and indications for spinal immobilization. It concludes with the statement that participants should follow their protocols and discuss such items with their medical director prior to changing their practices.

Skill Station 1—Patient Assessment "A"

The four participants are separated into two teams, with one team doing the assessment and the other team observing. Then the teams switch roles and the process is repeated. Each of the four participants will be a team leader in either this station or in the second assessment station. Using a scenario that presents a patient with simple trauma, the instructor sees the participants perform, in proper priority and sequence, a primary examination (including an initial global survey followed by a more in-depth A B C D E); follows that examination with the determination that initiation of rapid transport is not indicated; and performs a thorough head-to-foot secondary survey. The assessment steps are actually performed, but interventions and treatments are only verbalized. The instructor remediates problems found in the participants' assessment.

Skill Station 2—Patient Assessment "B"

As in Assessment Station "A," the four participants are divided into two teams of two members and the assessment is performed by each team. Each of the four participants is to be the team leader once in *either* Assessment Station "A" or Assessment Station "B." Using a scenario that presents a patient with multisystem trauma who is severely compromised, the instructor sees the participants perform the primary survey; identify critical injuries/conditions and verbalize the needed interventions; identify in no more that 3 to 4 minutes that the rapid initiation of transport is necessary; verbalize the rapid packaging and initiation of transport; verbalize the needed continued key treatments en route; and perform a rapid secondary survey en route as time and the patient's other needs allow. The assessment steps are actually performed, but interventions and treatments are only verbalized. The instructor remediates problems found in the participants' assessment.

Skill Station 3—Airway and Ventilation

All participants, both basic and advanced, demonstrate their ability to perform the trauma jaw thrust (alone) and the trauma chin lift with an assistant; to direct an assistant in providing immobilization; to measure and insert an oropharyngeal and a nasopharyngeal airway; and to provide a proper minute volume with a bag-valve-mask device while an assistant provides manual immobilization. Upon questioning from the instructor, participants demonstrate their understanding that initial ventilations may have to be started with room air, but that as rapidly as possible a collector or reservoir device attached to a high-flow oxygen source should be added. Each of the four participants demonstrates these skills in turn and is remediated by the instructor as needed.

Skill Station 4—Advanced Airway and Thoracentesis

[Advanced Course Refresher Participants Only]

With an assistant to help provide immobilization, advanced participants demonstrate their ability to perform visualized orotracheal intubation and blind nasotracheal intubation. The instructor, by questioning, determines the participants' understanding of the indication and possible contraindications of these procedures. Finally, on a manikin or model participants demonstrate their ability to establish the proper equipment and landmarks for needle thoracentesis and an understanding of the indication for the procedure and how to perform the procedure. Each participant in turn demonstrates each skill and is remediated as needed by the instructor.

Skill Station 5—Spine Skills "A"
Logrolls and Standing Longboard

Working as a team, participants demonstrate a proper logroll for a supine-presenting patient; a proper logroll for a semiprone-presenting patient including an understanding of when the cervical collar should be applied; and a rapid standing longboard maneuver. The instructor will provide remediation as required. The instructor will question participants regarding the standing longboard technique used with stable patients to assure that they understand the affixation and sequence for this method.

Skill Station 6—Spine Skills "B"
Rapid Extrication

Working as a team, participants demonstrate their ability to perform a rapid extrication of a multisystem trauma patient sitting in a car. Participants will use manual immobilization techniques to rotate and lower the patient onto the longboard and remove him or her to a safe distance for the rapid institution of intervention. The instructor remediates as needed.

Written Examination

Procedure for the written examination follows the same recommendations established by the National Association of Emergency Medical Technicians Prehospital Trauma Life Support Program.

MECHANICS, EQUIPMENT, AND PERSONNEL

Faculty Needed for the Refresher Course

In addition to the PHTLS refresher course faculty, a course will also need the following: two to six lecturers, six skill station instructor/evaluators (or 12 if class size dictates two of each station, etc.), and a proctor for the written test. An assistant to help with the assembly and distribution of equipment for the skill stations is helpful.

Lecturers and skill station instructor/evaluators do not need to be present for the entire course. Skill station instructor/evaluators should be present for the entire 3 hours and, if needed, the time shown in the schedule for individual post-skill-station remediation as needed.

Selection of Lecturers

There are six lectures in the PHTLS refresher course. Use of at least two lecturers, for a varied presentation, is required. The total number of lecturers to be used for each course is based on the preference of the course coordinator and course medical director. Experience shows that three or four generally affords the best dynamics.

The PHTLS affiliate faculty shall give the course purpose presentation. He or she may also be scheduled to present other lectures at the option of the course medical director and course coordinator. As with the PHTLS provider courses, this individual is also prepared to present any of the lectures if a scheduled speaker cancels on the day of the course.

Lecture faculty should be selected on the basis of their understanding and acceptance of the concepts of the PHTLS program, their prehospital related experience, and their ability to present the material. As with the PHTLS provider course, individuals with strong prehospital orientation and experience are generally favored over those with strictly in-hospital clinical experience.

The selection of the lecturer presenting "Megatrends in Trauma" needs to be made carefully because this presentation should be expected to generate a significant number of questions about the state-of-the-art and local policy. This lecturer needs to be knowledgeable in current controversies, familiar with the prevailing current literature, and knowledgeable of the local protocols for that region. Although not required, it is recommended that this lecture be given by the course medical director, another emergency or trauma physician, or a paramedic course director/coordinator with such knowledge.

Selection of Skill Station Instructor/Evaluators

Because most refresher courses will have both basic and advanced participants, there will be six skill stations which run concurrently requiring a minimum of six skill station instructor/evaluators. Larger class sizes may require duplication of stations and enlarge this need to 12 or more individuals.

While it is preferred that PHTLS instructors run the various stations, the course coordinator and course medical director may assign qualified EMTs, emergency or critical care nurses, or emergency or trauma physicians to this task.

In courses containing advanced participants it is required that the instructor/evaluator for the assessment stations be trained to the advanced level and that the instructor/evaluator for the Advanced Airway Station (Station 4) be an EMT-paramedic, nurse, or PA with advanced airway and chest decompression training, or a physician.

Written Test Proctor

Procedure for selecting a written test proctor follows the same recommendations established by the National Association of Emergency Medical Technicians Prehospital Trauma Life Support Program.

FACILITIES, ROOMS, AND SETUP ────────

The setup of facilities and rooms follows the same recommendations established by the National Association of Emergency Medical Technicians Prehospital Trauma Life Support Program.

Six skill station rooms or areas (or more if in a larger course the skill stations are to be duplicated) will be needed. Each skill station should be large enough to accommodate four students, at least one evaluator, a victim, and all equipment necessary for the station, with sufficient additional room for free movement by the students as they perform the practical exercises. In cases where more than one station will be in the same room, some physical divider should be used to visually separate stations. The dividers should be a suitable distance from each other within the room to ensure that conversation in one station does not distract participants in another. Individual stations need to be identified and labeled with signs outside their entrances.

Spine Skills "B" Rapid Extrication (Station 6) requires a car and, in reasonable weather, is done outside. An alternate site should be identified (an equipment bay, under a hotel parapet, a maintenance garage, or an enclosed parking deck, etc.) for use in the event of rain or snow.

If lunch is provided, even for small courses, it needs to be prearranged with the cafeteria or food service personnel including lunch tickets, time, etc. The proximity of the eating facility to the other course activities is a consideration.

EQUIPMENT

The source of each piece of necessary equipment needs to be identified early in the planning process. Ideally, all of the equipment will be gathered in one place several days or a week before the course date so that the course coordinator is assured that all of the necessary equipment items have been obtained and that each is in proper working order. This allows time to obtain or replace missing, incorrect, or unusable items.

The equipment necessary for skill stations is detailed in two lists: a single cumulative integrated Master List/Combined Skills Station Equipment List for the course and separate equipment lists for individual stations. This will assist in planning and in setting up the skill stations. The lists by skill station are part of each skill station's outline.

PRECOURSE MAILING

Adequate promotion done well enough in advance of the course date is the key to maximizing enrollment. Experience has shown that when courses have obtained less than the desired number of participants it was most commonly because of inadequate promotion. Enrollment also suffered if the course presented a scheduling conflict with other local activities. With good planning, promotion can be done simply and inexpensively and does not require costly graphics.

The brochure should include:
- Host and sponsor citation
- Course location
- Course date
- Course prerequisites
- Mention of 3-year recognition period
- Course description and schedule
- Faculty information
- Name of the course medical director

- Map (where applicable)
- CEUs offered (CECBEMS)
- Course fee
- Additional cost if student needs a textbook
- A preregistration form
- A number to call for more information or to register by telephone

The preregistration section of the brochure (either returned by mail or filled out by the person taking a telephone preregistration) should include:
- Participant's name
- Current mailing address
- Phone/contact information
- Current level of certification
- Squad affiliation
- Which previous course(s) taken (PHTLS Basic, PHTLS Advanced, BTLS Basic, BTLS Advanced, PHTLS Refresher)
- When and where previous course(s) taken
- Name and edition of current PHTLS text including a statement that it is required, a space to check if one will be needed, and a price
- Statement regarding policy for students who cancel

Whether payment of the course fee is required with the application or at a later date is a matter of preference and should be determined by the course coordinator. If institutions or services will be paying for a group of participants, a purchase order often replaces the advance payment, with the actual payment being made after the course (once the "service" has been rendered).

A confirmation, welcome, and information letter should be sent to each preregistered participant.

The letter should include:
- A welcome
- Course dates and times
- The time participants will need to arrive for on-site course registration
- Where course will be held (name of facility and address)
- Precise location of course registration area: exact building, room, etc.
- Information regarding parking
- Information on clothing (comfortable, casual, etc.)
- Information on lunch availability, cost, etc.
- Indication check has been received *or* date by which payment must be received to hold registrant's space in course
- Acknowledgment that participants already have the text *or* date on which text will be sent or will be available for pickup
- A phone number or pager number at which participants can be called during the course in the event of an emergency at home
- Emphasize that the course will start on time.
- Note that participants are expected to review the PHTLS text prior to the course.
- Emphasize that participants MUST bring a copy of their current certification card and MUST bring a copy of their previous PHTLS or BTLS provider (or last refresher) course certificate (or card) or proof of such successful completion to the course.
- A final course schedule with faculty names (or a separate faculty list)

While creating the letter, you should consider the need for:
- Detailed "campus" map, if appropriate
- Larger scale map and directions, if there are out-of-town participants
- Information on hotels/motels and local dinner and breakfast places if there are out-of-town participants
- An evening emergency contact number, or pager number, for reaching the course coordinator if out-of-town participants should have a problem on arrival the evening before the course

FORMS YOU WILL NEED FOR YOUR COURSE

In this guide you will find the other forms and materials you will need to make copies of for the PHTLS refresher course.
- PHTLS Refresher Course Coordinator Schedule (this section)
    - (1 copy in advance)
- Student Registration/Refresher Course Skill Station Summary Sheet (Section V)
    - (copy/student)
- Summary Evaluation Form (Section V)
    - (copy/student)
- Written Test Answer Sheet (Section V)
    - (copy/student)
- Course Summary Report (Section V)
    - (1 copy at course)
- Final Course Roster Form (Section V)
    - (1 copy at course)

The lecture outlines and skill station materials are included in this section. **Note:** It is a good idea to make an extra copy of the material for each skill station to bring to the course, since it is not uncommon for skill station instructor/evaluators to arrive without their copy. Also you should bring this guide to the course so that you have the master copies to make additional copies of any forms if needed or to copy a lecture outline if a lecturer has to cancel due to a last minute emergency.

COORDINATOR SCHEDULE ACTIVITY FORM

The coordinator schedule activity form follows the same recommendations established by the National Association of Emergency Medical Technicians Prehospital Trauma Life Support Program. For further details please refer to Section V of this manual.

STUDENT REGISTRATION FORM

The student registration form follows the same recommendations established by the National Association of Emergency Medical Technicians Prehospital Trauma Life Support Program. For further details please refer to Section V of this manual.

WRITTEN TEST ANSWER SHEET

The written test answer sheet follows the same form established by the National Association of Emergency Medical Technicians Prehospital Trauma Life Support Program. For further details please refer to Section V of this manual.

ROSTER

The roster follows the same forms established by the National Association of Emergency Medical Technicians Prehospital Trauma Life Support Program. For further details please refer to Section V of this manual.

COURSE CONTENT

SKILL STATIONS AND WRITTEN TEST INSTRUCTIONS

[To be read to students at the beginning of the written test]

The questions on the written test that you are about to take are multiple choice and represent a random selection from the key content and topics covered in the PHTLS course. Successful completion of the PHTLS refresher course requires a grade of 75% or higher on the written test and demonstration of your ability to competently perform the skills included in each of the skill stations.

After completing the written test all participants will rotate through five skill stations:

Station 1—Patient Assessment "A"
Station 2—Patient Assessment "B"
Station 3—Airway and Ventilation
Station 5—Spine Skills "A" Logroll and Standing Longboard
Station 6—Spine Skills "B" Rapid Extrication

Advanced personnel *only* will go through Station 4, which includes visualized orotracheal intubation, blind nasal intubation, and chest decompression.

The skills stations are located (describe) _____.
You will rotate through the stations in groups of four. When you leave the written test, go to (location) _____ where (name) _____ will make up the group of four and assign you to your first skill station.

No specific time frame for completing each station has been set. Once your group has finished a station, return to (name or location) _____ _____ and your group will be sent to the next available station. NO CHANGES are to be made in the make-up of a group.

At each station the evaluator will provide specific instructions and ask you to demonstrate a particular skill or skills. The evaluator will offer any suggestions or remediations needed to ensure that you can perform the skills at a high level of competence before leaving the station.

In the event that additional remediation is needed in the station within a reasonable period of time, you will be required to return at the end of the day.

Any participant needing to retest on any stations or on the written test will have an opportunity for remediation and retesting in the time scheduled for that purpose at the end of the course.

[Give each student a copy of the written test, answer sheet, and his or her own registration form.]

If you turn the registration form over you will note that the back includes a place for the evaluators to note your progress through the skill stations. Be sure to have it filled in after each station and return it after your group has finished all of the stations. Please PRINT your name in the appropriate place at the top of this form, and PRINT your name, Social Security number, course location, and today's date at the top of the answer sheet.

Do not mark or write in the test booklet. Mark your answers on the answer sheet by blackening out or covering over the letter representing the answer you have selected. Be sure to answer all of the questions, and be careful to mark the correct number on the answer sheet for the question that you are answering.

You have until (time) _____ to complete the written test. Remember to keep your registration form when you turn in your test booklet and answer sheet. Take it with you to the skill stations.

INSTRUCTIONS FOR SKILL STATION EVALUATORS

Introduction

The skill station objectives for the refresher course are:
- to affirm the individual's ability to perform the skills competently
- to remediate individual performance of previously learned skills **as needed** to improve performance
- to identify groups or individuals who require additional instruction and reevaluation (beyond a reasonable amount of time in the station) at a later time in order to reach the required level of competence

All participants **should** be able to perform all of the required skills. Many will do this in an exemplary demonstration without need of any comment beyond "well done." Others will benefit from some suggestions or remediation of their technique. Care must be taken not to spend the additional time that "teaching" would require as this will cause a significant delay for other groups. Time has been scheduled for this at the end of the day.

After completing your station, you may be asked to stay and provide additional instruction for such students. At that time you should "teach" the skill and then evaluate their abilities after they have received this additional instruction.

Method

As participants finish the written test they will be organized into groups of four. **It is essential that you mark each student's form; this is the only record of his or her performance in your station.** The time needed to complete your station will vary from group to group, therefore unlike in most provider courses there are no preset periods for changing stations. **(However, no group should be allowed to take more than 30 minutes in any station.)**

If you have any questions about the procedure or your station, consult with the affiliate faculty or course coordinator for clarification before starting. If a question or problem occurs during the rotations, resolve it with the affiliate faculty prior to starting the next group.

Keep track of the number of groups that rotate through your station. This will assist you and the coordinator in knowing how many students still need to complete your station. At the end of the day we would appreciate your help in reassembling all of the equipment before you leave.

SKILL STATION 1—PATIENT ASSESSMENT "A"

Purpose

The purpose of this skill station is to affirm and, as needed, increase the participant's ability to perform a complete, thorough trauma assessment. In addition, the sequence should properly reflect the established priorities for identifying conditions requiring needed interventions.

The mechanism of injury in this station suggests the possibility of serious injury but, on examination, the moulaged patient is found to have only a variety of individual simple injuries which *do not* have any multisystem impact or resultant instability. After receiving the scenario and instructions, participants are expected to:
- evaluate the scene,
- perform a rapid global survey,
- perform the rest of the primary survey,
- perform a complete head-to-foot secondary survey,
- obtain a proper history, and
- verbalize the interventions and treatments indicated. This should include the timely identification that no immediate urgency exists in this patient, allowing for the secondary survey and individual item care and packaging to be accomplished at the scene.

Method

The participants arrive at the station in a group of four and are divided into two pairs of responders with a "leader" identified for each pair. The assessment is performed by both teams, one at a time. Each participant is to be a team leader once in either Station 1 or Station 2.

All steps in the assessment are to be done by the team leaders or on their direct order by the assisting EMT. Treatment is not actually provided, only verbalized.

Unlike a typical testing station where an unstable multisystem trauma patient is presented, this station's scenario is only used to set the stage and the patient remains stable.

The scenario is designed to promote the display of a complete thorough assessment without the need of urgent initiation of transport.

Equipment

Essential
Disposable examination gloves (1 pair per student)
Blood pressure cuff
Penlight
Stethoscope
Long backboard
1 model victim "patient"

Optional
PASG
4 backboard straps
2 blankets
Vest or 1/2 board spine device
Traction splint
4 cravats
2 towels
Rigid cervical collar (Stiff Neck, Philadelphia, or equivalent)

Airway Kit including:
Oral or nasal airway
Non-rebreather O_2 mask
Demand valve
BVM with reservoir

IV Kit including:
2 1000 ml bag RL or NS
Paper or adhesive tape
2 macrodrip tubing sets
IV constricting band

Moulage

The patient described in the scenario for this station is the driver of a motorcycle. He "laid the bike down," separating from it prior to the vehicle colliding with a van. His helmet is removed prior to the squad's arrival, and he is found wearing a long sleeve shirt, heavy jeans, and sturdy shoes or boots.

His injuries that should be moulaged are as follows:
Right shoulder—lateral to posterior bruise
Right mid-humerus—contusion
Right hand—minor lacerations, capillary ooze
Right thorax—assorted road rash laterally
Right hip—large contusion
Right leg—assorted road rash laterally
Right lower leg—large midshaft contusion

Directions to Be Read to the Participants
[Introduce yourself and collect each participant's Refresher Course Skill Station Summary Sheet.]
The purpose of this station is to see you perform a thorough assessment as you would in the field. You will go through this station in a team of two members. One of the members of each team will be the team leader and will be required to do the assessment. The second team member can assist with quantitative vital signs, etc. There will also be two imaginary EMT helpers who can perform interventions, get equipment, etc. All of the assessment steps need to be actually performed. Interventions and treatments need to be verbalized only, *not* actually performed. Any equipment normally found in an ambulance that is not here will be imagined to be present if required.

When you perform steps such as checking the skin, be sure to tell me what you are looking at. As you do your assessment, the patient or I will supply you with the pertinent findings. If at any time you lose your place, since this is not an actual patient, stop and ask me and I will recap the steps you have performed and your findings to that point.

NOTE: Now divide the group in two teams and identify the leader for each team. Make sure they understand that they should not leave the immediate area or go to another station. Then read the first team the following scenario. (After the first team is finished, repeat the scenario, and proceed with the second team.)

Scenario

Upon arrival at the scene you are told of and observe a 23-year-old male (adjust age and gender to fit model, but under 30 years of age, regardless) who had been traveling on a two-lane road at moderate speed. At an intersection, a van traveling on the cross street slowed at the stop sign, failed to come to a full stop, then proceeded into the intersection in front of the motorcycle. The motorcycle operator, realizing that he could not avoid colliding with the side of the van, slowed and then "laid down" the bike on its right side.

After the driver separated from it, the motorcycle slid forward and struck the rear corner of the van—no fire or explosion occurred. The van driver is uninjured. Police officers at the scene confirm that nobody else is injured. The motorcycle operator is found supine on the ground about 15 feet from the van and motorcycle. His helmet has been removed prior to your arrival, and he is wearing heavy blue jeans, a long-sleeve flannel shirt, and sturdy shoes. It is a nice sunny day, temperature about 78° F.

Checklist for Use During Skill Station

Patient has:
- Contusion right shoulder (sprain/strain)
- Contusion right midshaft humerus (closed fracture)
- Minor contusions and lacerations right hand
- "Road rash" right lateral thorax
- Contusion right hip (rule out fracture/dislocation)
- "Road rash" lateral right leg
- Contusion midshaft right lower leg (closed fracture)

- Skin is pale, cool, and moist (mild early compensated shock).
- Pulse—88, strong and regular
- Blood pressure—120/80
- Ventilations—24 and regular
- Patient is alert and oriented (A&O ×3).
- Patient is anxious about motorcycle but NOT argumentative or combative.
- Chief complaints: Severe pain to right upper arm, right hip, and right lower leg
- Pain on palpation/movement, right shoulder, right upper arm, right hand, right midthorax (R5), right hip, and right leg.
- Upon auscultation, breath sounds are present bilaterally, are symmetrical, and indicate an adequate tidal volume. Heart sounds are normal.
- Abdomen is soft and normal. Pelvis is intact and normal except for pain at contusion in right hip area.
- Pupils are equal, round, and react to light.
- Motor ability, sensory response, and circulation are present in all four extremities. Patient guards against movement of right arm or right leg due to pain.
- History reveals no loss of consciousness, nor alcohol, or drugs. Ate lunch 1 hour prior to collision. No known allergies. No pertinent medical history.

Patient does not deteriorate regardless of care provided. With proper care (basic shock treatment with oxygen and careful examination), the vital signs when rechecked become:

Pulse—78
Blood pressure—120/76
Ventilations—20
Skin pink, warm, and dry
Patient calms

Outline of Care

- Evaluates scene and situation
- Ensures body surface isolation (BSI)
- Evaluates number of victims/resources needed
- Orders/provides manual immobilization of head
- Identifies self, elicits history and chief complaint
- Performs rapid global survey (evaluates gross LOC, ventilation, shock, hemorrhage)
- Proceeds to a more detailed primary (A B C D)
- Checks airway/mouth
- Check neck (bruises, wounds, JVD, tracheal deviation, subcutaneous emphysema)
- Orders/applies cervical collar
- Observes, palpates, auscultates chest (breath and heart sounds)
- Observes, palpates abdomen; checks pelvis
- Takes/orders other to take vital signs
- AVPU, evaluates if any period of unconsciousness occurred postincident and determines present level of alertness and orientation
- Assesses PEARL and consensual reflex
- Checks ears, nose, mouth for fluid, Battle's sign, and "raccoon eyes"

- Checks motor ability, sensory response, and circulation in all four extremities
- Evaluates and identifies that patient is stable. Rules out possibility of multisystem trauma
- Performs head-to-toe secondary survey
- Locates all injuries (as described)
- Obtains AMPLE (or greater) past history
- Verbalizes appropriate shock care
- Verbalizes that patient is immobilized to longboard
- Verbalizes appropriate wound and fracture care
- (Advanced personnel only) Verbalizes IV consideration (NOTE: may determine none needed, or one or two lines established at TKO/KVO rate)
- Verbalizes packaging and initiation of transport
- Verbalizes simulated radio report

Be sure to initial the participants' Refresher Course Skill Station Summary Sheet to indicate their performance in this station, and return the sheet to them before they leave your station.

Purpose

The purpose of this skill station is to affirm and increase the participant's ability to perform a complete thorough assessment on a severely compromised trauma patient in a sequence that properly reflects accepted priorities for identifying/ruling out conditions and providing needed intervention. In this station the patient is a multisystem trauma patient with compromised ventilation and circulation and a greatly reduced level of consciousness.

After receiving the scenario and instructions, the participants are expected to:
- Evaluate the scene,
- Perform a rapid global survey,
- Perform the rest of the primary survey,
- Identify the need to rapidly package and transport,
- Continue providing key interventions en route,
- Obtain a proper history, and
- Verbalize that if time and resources allow, they would perform a secondary survey while en route.

Method

The participants arrive at the station in a group of four and are divided into two pairs of responders with a "leader" identified for each pair. The assessment is performed by both teams, one at a time. Each participant is to be a team leader once in either station 1 or station 2.

All steps in the assessment are to be done by the team leader or on his or her direct order by the assisting EMT. Treatment is not actually provided, only verbalized.

As in a classical testing station, conditions that are properly identified and treated improve, while conditions that are not identified or not properly treated produce the appropriate deterioration. Because even with moulage a visual difference exists between the stimulus provided in a mock patient and a real one, the evaluator should volunteer and reinforce any information (pallor, diaphoresis, dyspnea, etc.) that would be globally apparent on a real patient at any step in the examination.

SKILL STATION 2—PATIENT ASSESSMENT "B"

Once the team is "en route" to the hospital with the patient, have "started" IVs and rechecked vital signs, and are beginning a detailed head-to-foot secondary examination, the evaluator indicates that the team has arrived at the hospital and that the team has noted that the secondary examination would have been done if time allowed.

Equipment

Disposable examination gloves (1 pair/student)
Blood pressure cuff
Penlight
Stethoscope
Long backboard
1 moulaged model victim "patient"
PASG
6 backboard straps
1 blanket
Vest or 1/2 board spine device
Traction splint
4 cravats
2 towels
Rigid cervical collar (Stiff Neck, Philadelphia, or equivalent)

Airway Kit including:
Oral airway
Nasal airway
Non-rebreather O_2 mask
Demand valve
BVM with reservoir

IV kit including:
2 1000 ml bag RL or NS
Paper or adhesive tape
2 macrodrip tubing sets
IV constricting band

NOTE: Because treatments and interventions are only verbalized, participants will actually use only the examining gloves, BP cuff, stethoscope, penlight, and possibly the long backboard. Although not actually used, the remaining items listed above should be evident and available in the station to serve as visual clues by their presence. For example, when a C-collar is ordered, place it on; when IVs are "started", tape the tubing to the site; when PASG is ordered, lay the garment over the abdomen, legs, etc.

Moulage

The multisystem trauma patient described in the scenario for this station is a construction worker who fell off a scaffolding to the ground from a height of approximately 10 feet and landed on some construction materials. He is found supine on the ground. He has severely compromised ventilation and is in decompensated shock. He speaks with guarded difficulty and is not sure of the events of the accident.

The conditions and injuries that should be moulaged are as follows:
  Left forehead—small contusion
  Face skin—white-grayish, marked diaphoresis
  Left anterior midthorax—large linear contusion
  Left upper quadrant of abdomen—large linear contusion (midthorax and abdomen from wheelbarrow)
  Left wrist—significant contusion (closed fracture)
  Left ankle—significant contusion (closed fracture)
  Right lower leg, midshaft—contusion and deformity (closed fracture)

Directions to Be Read to the Participants
[Introduce yourself and collect each participant's Refresher Course Skill Station Summary Sheet.]
The purpose of this station is to see you perform a thorough assessment as you would in the field. You will go through this station in a team of two members. One of the members of each team will be the team leader and will be required to do the assessment. The second team member can assist with quantitative vital signs, etc. There will also be two imaginary EMT helpers who can perform interventions, get equipment, etc. All of the assessment steps need to be actually performed. Interventions and treatments need to be verbalized only, *not* actually performed. The normal equipment from the ambulance typical of what might be needed for use with a real patient is provided in the station to assist you with its "visual" presence. If you wish, you may apply items on the patient (such as the PASG) to remind you where you are or what you have done so far.

When you perform steps such as checking the skin, be sure to tell me what you are looking at. As you do your assessment, the patient or I will supply you with the pertinent findings. If at any time you lose your place, since this is not an actual patient, stop and ask me and I will recap the steps you have performed and your findings to that point.

NOTE: Now divide the group in two teams and identify the leader for each team. Make sure they understand that they should not leave the immediate area or go to another station. Then read the first team the following scenario. (After the first team is finished, repeat the scenario, and proceed with the second team.)

Scenario

When you arrive at the scene you note that it is the site of a 3-story office building under construction. You are directed to the side of the building where you see a scaffolding in place with a platform about 10 feet above the ground. The ground is typical of a construction site: pieces of equipment, piles of debris, and mounds of earth are near the building's wall. The foreman meets you and says, "It's bad—he fell off the scaffold." The foreman was alerted by the victim's scream as he fell and saw him land on a wheelbarrow then slide off it to the ground. "I didn't let anyone move him," the foreman goes on to say.

Several others working nearby saw the victim fall and confirm the information given to you by the foreman. It is a warm sunny day, about 80°. A 32-year-old male (match age and sex to actual patient model) is found supine on a flat area of ground next to the wheelbarrow a few feet away from the base of the scaffolding.

Checklist for Use During Skill Station

Patient has:

 Small contusion on forehead
 Major linear contusion left midthorax with underlying pneumothorax or hemothorax (but not tension)
 Marked dyspnea
 Major linear contusion left upper quadrant of abdomen and fractured pelvis with intra-abdominal bleeding
 Profound decompensated shock
 Closed fracture of left wrist
 Closed fracture of left ankle
 Midshaft closed fracture of right tibia and fibula

- Skin is white-grayish and waxy in appearance and cold.
- Marked diaphoresis.
- Patient responds verbally in short two-word replies (with marked dyspnea).
- Patient's replies are appropriate but slowed, and he is unclear about what happened except that he fell. He knows his name, that he was working on a scaffold, and what day it is, but he is also anxious and confused in keeping with his levels of pain and shock.
- Pulse—peripheral pulses are *not* palpable
- Capillary refill time is slow—4 to 6 seconds
- Blood pressure—60/40
- Ventilations—36, shallow, marked dyspnea, and short of breath (SOB)
- Chief complaints—hurts all over, cannot breathe, weakness
- Pain on palpation/movement—forehead, left midthorax, LUQ, left wrist, left ankle, right lower leg (midshaft)
- Marked deformity and crepitus are found at left wrist, left ankle, and right lower leg.
- Neck veins are flat (normal for supine hypotensive patient).
- Trachea is midline.
- *No* subcutaneous emphysema is present.
- Chest has marked linear contusion in left midthorax from striking wheelbarrow. There is almost no left-sided chest movement on inspiration.
- Breath sounds on left are ABSENT when auscultated. Breath sounds on right are present but at 36/min and shallow.
- Heart sounds are normal.
- Abdomen has significant linear contusion across LUQ (from wheelbarrow) and is distended and rigid.
- Pelvis is found to be unstable and crepitus is present when stressed.
- Pupils are equal, round, and react to light with normal consensual reflex, but with slowed response.

- No fluid or blood is found at the nose, ear, or mouth. No indication of Battle's sign or "raccoon eyes"
- Motor ability and sensory response are present in all four extremities; however, movement is guarded in the three extremities with fractures. Distal circulation is ABSENT in all four extremities initially due to profound shock.
- History reveals that patient is unclear about events immediately after the fall: "I remember falling—then lots of pain." (Loss of time continuity = loss of consciousness). No alcohol; no drugs or medications. Last meal about 2 hours prior to incident. Previous allergic reaction to penicillin produced hives and shortness of breath. Previous fracture to left ankle about 2 years ago with unremarkable recovery to full use. No other pertinent medical history.

Outline of Care

- Evaluates scene and situation (including mechanism)
- Evaluates number of victims, resources needed
- Ensures body surface isolation (BSI)
- Orders/provides manual immobilization of head
- Identifies self, elicits history and chief complaint
- Performs rapid global survey (evaluates gross LOC, ventilation, shock, hemorrhage, speech ability, implementation)
- Proceeds to more detailed primary (A B C D)
- Checks airway/mouth
- Checks neck (bruises, wounds, JVD, tracheal deviation, subcutaneous emphysema)
- Orders/applies C-collar
- Observes, palpates, auscultates chest (breath and heart sounds)
- Observes, palpates abdomen
- Palpates/stresses pelvis
- Takes/orders others to take quantitative vital signs
- AVPU, evaluates a period of unconsciousness occurred postincident and determines present levels of alertness and orientation
- Checks ears, nose, mouth for blood or fluid and for Battle's sign and "raccoon eyes"
- Checks motor ability, sensory response, and peripheral circulation at some time in the examination to determine/rule out any neurologic deficit or limb-threatening circulatory compromise
- Obtains AMPLE (or greater) past history
- Locates key conditions/injuries with systemic implication (pneumothorax, intra-abdominal hemorrhage, fractured pelvis, potentially unstable spine)
- Identifies that patient has multisystem trauma
- Rapidly initiates packaging and transport without delay
- Verbalizes immobilization to longboard
- Radios hospital to alert them of inbound multisystem trauma patient

Key treatments ordered/verbalized were:
- Manages airway (manual to adjuncts, prn)
- Evaluates/provides adequate minute volume (BVM)
- Provide FiO$_2$ of 0.85 or greater
- Provides proper care for shock/abdominal bleeding
- (Advanced personnel) Provides proper fluid replacement and cardiac monitoring while en route

 – Provides proper immobilization (spine and other musculoskeletal injuries)

Be sure to initial the participants' Refresher Course Skill Station Summary Sheet to indicate their performance in this station, and return the sheet to them before they leave your station.

SKILL STATION 3—AIRWAY AND VENTILATION

Purpose

The purpose of this skill station is to affirm and, as needed, increase the participant's ability to properly manage/secure the airway of a trauma victim with manual maneuvers and simple adjuncts and to provide ventilation at a proper rate and volume with a bag-valve-mask device while manual immobilization of the patient's head in the neutral, in-line position is maintained throughout.

Method

Using an intubation head or other airway training manikin, each participant will perform the following skills:
 – trauma jaw thrust
 – trauma chin lift
 – measure and insert an oropharyngeal airway using either the tongue-jaw lift or tongue-blade method
 – measure and insert a nasopharyngeal airway

Each of these skills (except the trauma jaw thrust) is performed with an assistant maintaining manual, in-line immobilization. The trauma jaw thrust is to be done without an assistant by each participant while simultaneously maintaining the neutral immobilization of the head.

Each participant is also to demonstrate his or her ability to ventilate the "patient" at a rate of 16 to 24 times per minute at a volume (estimated) of 800 ml/breath or greater. This is to be done while the participant maintains immobilization and mask seal as well as when an assistant is available to maintain the immobilization and mask seal, leaving both of the participant's hands free to deflate the bag.

The importance of initiating ventilation of the apneic patient in under 30 seconds (with room air *or* high FiO_2) and ultimately with high FiO_2 as soon as possible is reviewed. Indications, contraindications, and the preferred or required position of the operator for each method and device is asked and reviewed.

Each of the skills in this station are detailed and discussed in the current PHTLS text and should be carefully reviewed by the evaluator prior to the course.

Equipment

Essential

Adult intubation manikin or equivalent airway/ventilation training device
Disposable gloves (1 pair/student)

Nasopharyngeal airway (correct size for manikin)
Oropharyngeal airway (correct size for manikin)
Tongue blades
Bag-valve-mask device with adult mask, reservoir, and oxygen connect-
ing tubing

Optional
Rigid cervical collar
Oxygen tank with regulator and key
Nasopharyngeal airways (various sizes)
Oropharyngeal airways (various sizes)

Directions to Be Read to the Participants
*[Introduce yourself and collect each participant's Refresher Course Skill
Station Summary Sheet.]*
The purpose of this station is to perform the trauma jaw thrust and trauma
chin lift, measure and insert an oropharyngeal airway, measure and insert a
nasopharyngeal airway, and to ventilate the patient at a proper rate and volume using a bag-valve-mask device both alone and with an assistant. Each
of these is to be performed maintaining manual immobilization of the head
in the neutral, in-line position. This station is *not* done as a scenario-based
progression.

Checklist for Use During Skill Station

**Indicate that the manual trauma airway maneuvers (trauma jaw thrust and
trauma chin lift) will be done first.**

Trauma Jaw Thrust

– Ask what the advantage is of the trauma jaw thrust over the trauma
chin lift. (Can be performed with immobilization by a single operator)
– Ask the participant to perform the maneuver.
– Ensures body surface isolation (BSI)
– Positions self above (beyond) patient's head facing caudally (see note
below)
– Grasps patient's head with fingers at side, thumbs on face. Places/
maintains head in neutral, in-line position
– With fourth and fifth fingers under the angles of the mandible, moves
the mandible anteriorly (and slightly caudally to open mouth) until the
lower jaw is noticeably extended
– Head does not move
– Repeat maneuver with each patient

Note and discuss that this maneuver can be done either from beyond the
patient's head facing caudally and with the fingers pointing caudally, or it
can be done from beside the chest, facing the patient's head with the fingers
pointing cephalad.

Trauma Chin Lift

**Instruct an assistant to provide manual immobilization of the head from
above (beyond) the patient's head.**
– Ask the participant to perform the maneuver.
– Ensures body surface isolation (BSI)

- Grasps chin between thumb and first two fingers at the midline
- Places other hand on patient's forehead (optional)
- Pulls the chin anteriorly and slightly caudally, elevating the mandible and opening the mouth. (The tongue-jaw lift with the thumb inserted in the mouth is *not* acceptable. It does not allow for a mask seal when ventilating and should only be temporarily used to insert a device in an unresponsive patient.)
- Repeat maneuver with each participant.

Oropharyngeal Airway

- Ask what would contraindicate use of an oropharyngeal airway. (Intact gag reflex)
- Instruct an assistant to provide manual immobilization

Tongue-Jaw Lift Insertion Method

- Ask the participant to perform the maneuver.
- Ensures body surface isolation (BSI)
- Measures length (lower ear to corner of mouth)
- With one hand, performs tongue-jaw lift
- With other hand, holds oropharyngeal airway at a right angle to the long axis of the body
- With distal tip pointing posteriorly and slightly laterally, inserts tip superior to the tongue
- Advances airway into oropharynx allowing or helping it to rotate medially and to follow the normal curve of the patient's airway
- Continues advancing until the flanged end lies just anterior to the lips
- Releases tongue-jaw lift
- Ask participant what he or she would do if the patient gags at any time during the insertion.
- Repeat maneuver with each participant.

Tongue Blade Insertion Method

- Ask the participant to perform the maneuver.
- Ensures body surface isolation (BSI)
- Measures length (lower ear to corner of mouth)
- With one hand, firmly grasps tongue blade and inserts it superior to the tongue just beyond half the tongue's length
- Angles tongue blade so that the distal tip is more caudad than the proximal end, depressing the tongue against the floor of the mouth
- Holds oropharyngeal airway in the other hand with a pencil-like grip just below the flange in alignment with the midline of the patient's body
- With the distal tip pointing posteriorly into the mouth, inserts the airway superior to the tongue blade
- Advances the airway following the anatomic curvature of the upper airway
- Continues advancing airway until the flanged end lies just anterior to the lips
- Releases pressure on tongue blade and withdraws it
- Repeat maneuver with each participant.

Indicate to participant that either method can be used in adults but that the tongue blade method is used with small children. In keeping with body surface isolation, it should be pointed out that the tongue blade method minimizes the possibility of accidentally piercing the EMT's glove and skin.

Nasopharyngeal Airway

- Ask the participants to perform the maneuver.
- Ensures body surface isolation (BSI)
- Ask what the indication is for use of the nasopharyngeal airway. (Absence of gag reflex; problem of insertion with oropharyngeal airway)
- Have an assistant provide manual immobilization from above (beyond) the patient's head.
- Have the participant measure (verbalizing measurement criteria) and insert airway.
- Examines nostrils; selects largest and least deviated
- Selects appropriate diameter (just smaller than selected nostril or patient's little finger)
- If variable lengths for a given diameter or an adjustable length nasopharyngeal airway are available, participant indicates length measurement sized from lower ear to outer corner of nose
- Verbalizes/lubricates distal tip
- Holds airway with pencil-like grip
- Explains/instructs patient
- Inserts into anterior nares
- Gently advances in a posterior direction (*not* superior)
- When approximately two-thirds inserted, participant assumes that assistant is performing jaw thrust and mandible is anteriorly elevated to ensure airway passes behind the posterior tongue
- Continues advancing airway until flange is at the anterior nares
- Ask the participant what he or she would do if patient gags:
  a. During insertion. (Encourage patient to swallow.)
  b. As last half inch or so is inserted. (Withdraw slightly until tolerated.)
- Repeat maneuver with each participant.

Bag-Valve-Mask Ventilation

(Bag-valve, mask, reservoir, connecting tubing, and oxygen tank should NOT be preassembled or turned on. Only the regulator and tank can be connected.)

- Ask what would indicate the need to provide ventilation for a patient. (Apnea, inadequate spontaneous minute volume from any cause such as that with a rate of under 10 or over 30, or possibly under 12 and over 20.)
- Ensures body surface isolation (BSI)
- Have the participant provide bag-valve-mask ventilation to the apneic "patient" just as he or she would if performing as the only provider present. An oropharyngeal airway has already been inserted.
- Assembles correct size mask to bag-valve unit
- Initiates ventilation within 30 seconds (room air or oxygen)
- Properly seals mask to face
- Maintains elevation of mandible and mask seal
- Ventilates at a rate of 16 to 24 per minute
- Properly deflates bag (squeezing it against own forearm, thigh, or thorax)
- Provides (estimated) greater than 800 ml per ventilation
- Visualizes (verbalizes) chest to determine peak inspiration

– Allows adequate time between inhalations for exhalation (1:3 ratio)
– Adds reservoir and supplemental high-flow oxygen
– *Does not* interrupt ventilation for greater than 30 seconds
– Verifies adequacy of ventilations by feel of bag
– Checks/verbalizes need to auscultate midlung fields to verify adequate ventilation
– While an assistant provides manual immobilization, have the participant ventilate with the BVM.
– Uses both hands to deflate the bag
– Ventilates at proper rate and volume
– Allows adequate time between inhalations for exhalation (1:3 ratio)
– Ensures body surface isolation (BSI)

ADDITIONAL NOTES FOR THE INSTRUCTOR REGARDING AIRWAY AND VENTILATION

NOTE 1: If limited personnel are available, ventilations should be initiated without delay. After the patient has been ventilated with room air for a minute or two, ventilations should be interrupted for no more than 30 seconds to attach the reservoir and oxygen supply to provide a higher FiO_2. If only one provider is available and it takes more than 30 seconds to add the adjuncts, ventilation should be reinstituted for a minute or two after every 30-second pause until all of the equipment is attached and working.

NOTE 2: Explain that very few people can consistently deliver 800 ml or greater by squeezing the BVM with only their hands. Therefore, to ensure a proper tidal volume, it is recommended that everyone squeeze the bag against their forearm, thigh, or thorax when forced to use a BVM without an assistant.

Be sure to initial the participant's Refresher Course Skill Station Summary Sheet to indicate their performance in this station, and return the sheet to them before they leave your station.

SKILL STATION 4—ADVANCED AIRWAY MANAGEMENT

Only participants who have successfully completed an Advanced PHTLS or Advanced BTLS course previously and are advanced-level responders should complete this station.

Purpose

The purpose of this station is to affirm and, as needed, increase the ability to ADVANCED level participants to perform:
– Visualized orotracheal intubation while maintaining manual, neutral, in-line immobilization
– Blind nasotracheal intubation while maintaining manual, neutral, in-line immobilization
– Chest decompression by performing a simulated emergency needle thoracostomy

Indications and contraindications for each procedure are discussed.

Method

Begin with a manikin on the floor that has an oropharyngeal airway correctly inserted and that is being ventilated (BVM) by an assistant. The manikin head is held in the neutral, in-line position by a second assistant. Each participant is to assemble and prepare the necessary equipment and perform visualized orotracheal intubation, maintaining the neutral alignment throughout. Following insertion of the tube, each participant is to check to verify proper placement.

Second, each participant is to perform blind nasotracheal intubation on a manikin which simulates a conscious breathing patient.

Finally, each participant is to demonstrate the proper technique for an emergency needle thoracostomy. Using a decompression manikin (when available) or a chest plate with palpable ribs overlaying an inner tube, each participant verbalizes/locates the correct site, properly inserts the catheter and needle, removes the needle, adds a one-way valve device, and verbalizes securing the catheter to the chest.

The indications and contraindications for each procedure are discussed. It is recommended that all participants in the group complete one skill, then all proceed to the second, then to the third.

Equipment

Disposable gloves (1 pair/student)
1 adult intubation manikin and 1 can silicone spray
Stethoscope

Oral Intubation Setup including:
Laryngoscope set with handle and batteries, including:
Straight and curved adult blades
10 ml syringe
Stylet
8.0, 7.0, 6.0 ET tubes (1 each)
Tongue blades
Oral airway (sized to manikin)
BVM with reservoir

Nasal Intubation Setup including:
Selected items from oral intubation setup list
Bag-valve device without mask (to attach to manikin bronchus to provide exhalation)
Sterile water (to create misting in nasotracheal tube)

Pleural Decompression Setup including:
#20 gauge IV catheters
Macrodrip IV tubing set
1000 ml bag IV fluid
Scissors
Heimlich valve or extra latex gloves for flutter valves
EITHER:
Tire inner tube, 2 cans Fix-A-Flat (or equivalent), roll of duct tape, and half-slab of meat ribs,

OR:
Manikin chest plate with palpable ribs, tire inner tube, 2 cans Fix-A-Flat (or equivalent)

Checklist for Use During Skill Station

(Indicate that visualized orotracheal intubation will be first)

Visualized Orotracheal Intubation (with In-Line Immobilization)

(With the intubation head on the floor and an oropharyngeal airway properly inserted, have one participant position him or herself at the manikin's thorax facing the head and provide manual, in-line immobilization. Have a second participant ventilate the patient with a BVM from directly above the patient's head while facing caudally. Indicate that an oropharyngeal airway has been inserted and that BVM ventilations are being provided with a high FiO₂.)

- Ask what contraindications, if any, exist for prehospital visualized orotracheal intubation. (Present gag reflex.)
- Ask the participant to perform the procedure, which includes directing the assistants as needed.
- Ensures body surface isolation (BSI)
- Auscultates lungs bilaterally to establish baseline
- Selects proper size endotracheal tube and checks that cuff holds air
- Checks laryngoscope, prepares equipment, and verbalizes lubricating distal end of ET tube
- Participant sits on ground and gently moves forward with one leg over each of the manikin's "arms" until the head can be secured by the participant's thighs
- Directs ventilator to hyperventilate manikin
- Directs ventilator to stop; removes oral airway
- Performs tongue-jaw lift, inserts laryngoscope properly
- Directs assistant to apply pressure over larynx (optional)
- Visualizes manikin vocal cords by leaning backward while extending laryngoscope blade caudally and upward
- Without causing manikin head or neck to move, advances endotracheal tube through vocal cords to proper depth
- Without releasing tube, removes stylet if used, inflates cuff, and removes syringe from one-way valve
- Directs assistant to begin bag-valve ventilation through tube
- Observes chest rise and auscultates over each lung
- Ask what should be heard. (Good breath sounds bilaterally)
- Auscultates/verbalizes auscultation over epigastrium for at least one or two ventilations
- Ask what should be heard. (*No* rushing air or bubbling sounds on inhalation)
- Secures/verbalizes securing endotracheal tube with tape or device
- Verbalizes periodic reauscultation of lungs
- Ask/discuss what EMT would assume/do if after intubation both chest rise and distinct bilateral breath sounds were absent or the sounds of rushing air or bubbling sounds were heard over the epigastrium with each ventilation.
- Change positions and roles and repeat station with each participant.

Blind Nasotracheal Intubation

Place manikin on table or floor and connect second bag-valve device to one of manikin's bronchi. Have one assistant provide manual, in-line immobilization from above the manikin's head. Indicate that patient has spontaneous ventilation but inadequate minute volume.

- Ensures body surface isolation (BSI)
- Ask participant to perform the procedure.
- Ask when (prehospital) this technique would be selected over visualized orotracheal intubation. (When the gag reflex is intact)
- Ask what contraindications exist for this technique.
- Auscultates breath sounds bilaterally
- Selects proper equipment; tests that cuff holds air
- Measures and selects proper size endotracheal tube (just smaller than patient's anterior nares or diameter of little finger)
- Visualizes nostrils, selects least deviated
- Verbalizes lubricating tube
- Instructs patient
- Inserts tube into selected nostril, carefully advancing it posteriorly (Not superiorly)
- When approximately 1/3 of tube has been inserted, stops advancing tube and confirms/directs assistant to provide jaw-thrust to elevate tongue
- Visualizes misting of tube and rotates tube back and forth slowly to locate position where breath sounds are strongest and misting is greatest
- Gently advances tube into trachea to correct depth so that the cuff is beyond the vocal cords
- Without releasing the tube, inflates the cuff and removes the syringe from the one-way valve
- Ensures continued ventilations by observing chest rise and initially confirms proper placement by feeling air exchange at the external tube (not around it)
- Secondly, confirms proper placement by auscultation of lungs bilaterally and over epigastrium
- Verbalizes/secures tube with tape
- Change positions and roles and repeat with each participant.

Chest Decompression (Emergency Needle Thoracostomy)

Each of the steps in identifying the site and decompressing the chest are preferably performed on a manikin designed for the procedure. When such equipment is not available, an alternative device can be arranged using a manikin chest plate with palpable ribs taped over an inner tube which has been charged with Fix-A-Flat or similar tire-sealing substance.

- Ask what the indications are for chest decompression.
- Review that when a tension pneumothorax occurs in a patient in which a sucking wound has been sealed with an occlusive dressing, chest decompression should first be attempted by opening the occlusive dressing to release the tension ("burping" it).
- Identify the first participant who will do the needle decompression (or who will locate the site and verbalize the insertion and ensuing steps).
- Identifies presence of tension pneumothorax
- Ensures body surface isolation (BSI)
- Correctly identifies side and prepares necessary equipment

- With fingers of one hand, locates second or third intercostal space at the midclavicular line
- Cleanses skin with alcohol or other antiseptic solution
- Inserts large bore needle into thorax, sliding it over the top curve of the lower rib
- Once needle is inserted, carefully holds catheter hub to avoid kinking of the catheter and removes the needle
- Indicates that a rush of air is heard when the needle is removed
- Attaches a one-way valve (Heimlich valve or flutter valve made from latex glove finger, or IV tubing run to placement under water in a container placed at a height two or three feet lower on the floor)
- Secures/verbalizes securing catheter
- Auscultates chest bilaterally
- Rechecks/directs recheck of vital signs
- Change positions and roles and repeat with each participant.

Be sure to initial the participants' Refresher Course Skill Station Summary Sheet to indicate their performance in this station, and return the sheet to them before they leave your station.

SKILL STATION 5—SPINE SKILLS "A" LOGROLLS AND STANDING LONGBOARD

Purpose

The purpose of this station is to affirm and, as needed, improve the participants' ability to:

- logroll a supine patient onto a longboard
- logroll a semiprone patient to a supine position on a longboard
- immobilize an unstable standing patient to a longboard while lowering him or her to the ground

Each task is performed with manual immobilization of the head, neck, torso, and pelvis in the neutral, in-line position in order to keep movement of the spine to a minimum.

Method

Each of the skills is to be performed once by the four participants working together as a group. The station is not scenario-based or developmental. Each skill is done separately and solely as an isolated skill. For each of the skills, a different participant should serve as team leader, and the other participants should rotate roles so that the same person is not always holding the head, etc. The rapid standing longboard maneuver is used by participants for the standing patient immobilization; the alternative method wherein the patient is strapped to the board before lowering is discussed but not actually performed. By having the one person in the group who has not served as team leader describe that procedure, each participant will be highlighted once. Remediate any inadequacies or suggest changes to improve the group's performance. When possible, a live model should be used or have a participant rotate through this role.

Equipment

Essential
Longboard
Rigid cervical collar

Optional
Live model
Commercial head immobilizer or 2 blankets
6 backboard straps or cravats
3-inch tape or equivalent

Directions to Be Read to the Participants
[Introduce yourself and collect each participant's Refresher Course Skill Station Summary Sheet.]
In this station you will be asked as a group to logroll a supine patient onto a longboard, a semiprone patient onto a longboard, and to immobilize a standing patient to a longboard and lower him or her to a supine position on a longboard using the rapid method recommended for an unstable patient.

The station is not scenario-based. Each of the skills will be performed solely as isolated skills. In each case it has been established that the scene is safe and that no need for hemorrhage control or any other urgent intervention is required. Also, no patient condition exists which would hinder or cause you to alter any of the procedures you are being asked to perform. Please perform the maneuver as you would with a real patient.

After completing the three skills, I will ask the fourth member of your group to describe the steps in affixing a stable standing patient to the longboard prior to lowering it. In that way each of you will be placed in the leadership position at least once. As leaders change with each skill, be sure that the rest of you change positions each time also.

Checklist for Use During Skill Station

Logroll—Supine Patient
Indicate that the first maneuver will be logrolling a supine patient onto a longboard. When a participant is serving as a patient, indicate that you are available to place the longboard.
- Ask participant to perform the maneuver.
- Ensures body surface isolation (BSI)
- Directs one EMT to move patient's head to neutral, in-line position and maintain manual immobilization throughout
- Verbalizes checking: ABCs, MSC × 4, and neck
- Applies/directs application of rigid cervical collar
- Directs to which side the patient will be rolled
- Second EMT is positioned alongside patient's thorax.
- Third EMT is positioned alongside patient's knees.
- Patient's arms are placed against his or her sides with palms in and elbows "locked."
- Legs are grasped together with one hand or arm and moved to midline position.
- Longboard is placed next to patient on side opposite EMTs.
- EMTs at sides place their hands properly.

- Leader asks if all are ready; checks same
- Patient is rolled onto his or her side and perpendicular to the ground. The patient's feet are held about 4 to 6 inches off the ground to keep his or her legs parallel to the ground. The patient's head is maintained in a neutral, in-line position.
- Longboard is inserted (either held at 30° to 40° angle against the patient's lower side or on ground against patient's side or flat against patient's back according to the group's preference.
- Patient is lowered to the board in the same manner that was used to roll him or her. (If board was angled or upright, then patient and board are lowered to the ground.)
- With cervical alignment maintained, patient is centered on board as needed.
- Team leader verbalizes that patient would be immobilized to board and then ABCs and MSC × 4 rechecked.

Checklist for Use During Skill Station

Logroll—Semiprone Patient
Identify the maneuver and the participant who will act as team leader. When a participant is serving as a patient, indicate that you are available to place the longboard.

NOTE: This maneuver can be done in two ways depending on the placement of the longboard. Either the board can initially be placed on the ground next to the patient with the EMTs kneeling on it, or the board can be inserted along the patient's back once the patient has been logrolled perpendicular to the ground. The following steps include both methods. The participant serving as team leader should choose which method he or she wishes to have the group perform.

- Instruct the team leader to perform the maneuver.
- Ensures body surface isolation (BSI)
- Directs one EMT to hold the head, immobilizing it in the position found and holding it in such a way as to anticipate rolling the patient
- Directs check of airway and breathing
- Directs alignment of patient's arms and legs
- Rapidly checks patient's back for injuries and foreign objects
- Directs placing board alongside patient on the side opposite of the way he or she is facing. Board is to be 4 to 6 inches away from patient.
- Second EMT kneels on the longboard at the patient's thorax and properly grasps patient by holding patient's arms at his or her side with the elbows "locked."
- Third EMT kneels on the longboard and properly places one hand at the patient's hip and holds the patient's legs together at the ankles with his or her other hand.
- Team leader asks if all are ready; checks same
- On command, patient is rolled until he or she is perpendicular to the ground. The patient's head is rotated less than the torso into the neutral, in-line position. Patient's legs are maintained in neutral, in-line position with the feet elevated above the ground 3 to 5 inches.
- Directs insertion of longboard on its edge alongside the patient's back
- (BOTH OPTIONS)
- Directs EMT at thorax to shuffle backwards on his or her knees without moving the patient (to allow space for continuing the logroll to the ground)

- Once the EMT at the chest has finished moving backwards, gives same direction to EMT at the legs
- Asks if all are ready; checks same
- On command, logroll of patient (or patient and board) is continued in the same direction as before until patient and board are on the ground.
- Applies/directs application of rigid cervical collar (cannot be done earlier)
- Without loss of in-line immobilization, patient is centered on board.
- Verbalizes that group would provide appropriate interventions, immobilize patient to longboard, and recheck ABCs and MSC × 4.

NOTE: Acknowledge the method selected to be a good option, then discuss the other option to ensure that the participants are familiar with both procedures and understand that the selection of one or the other is based upon individual preference or may be dictated by the amount of space at the scene or by the type of backboard available.

Checklist for Use During Skill Station

Standing Longboard Application—Unstable Patient
Identify the maneuver and the participant who will be the team leader. If a participant will be used as the patient, select the smallest and lightest participant available (not the team leader) and indicate that you will be available to assist in stepping the board as directed.
- Direct the team leader to perform the maneuver.
- Ensures body surface isolation (BSI)
- Directs EMT to provide manual, in-line immobilization while standing behind the patient
- Directs second EMT to support patient by holding his or her thorax or under armpits
- Directs third EMT to insert longboard behind patient
- EMT behind patient lifts his or her elbows to allow board to be inserted. When it is in place, EMT presses the board against the patient's back.
- Directs second and third EMTs to take positions slightly anterior and at each side of the patient at an angle facing the patient
- Each EMT at the side inserts his or her hand under the patient's armpit and grasps the nearest backboard handhold ABOVE the armpit and presses against the patient's arm so that it cannot elevate.
- EMTs at the side then grasp a handhold near the top of the board with their free hand.
- Directs fourth team member (or evaluator) to "step" the bottom of the board
- Directs lowering of head end of the board part way to the ground and then stops the lowering.
- The EMT holding the head rotates one hand and then the other (moving fingers from pointing anterior to caudad).
- Each EMT in turn repositions his or her hand so that it will free the arms of the EMT who is holding the head when lowering is continued.
- Asks if all are ready to continue lowering; checks same
- On command, EMTs lower the board to the ground. The EMT at the head goes from standing to kneeling.
- Directs/assures continued manual immobilization of the head
- Applies/directs application of rigid cervical collar
- Verbalizes that assessment, needed interventions, and mechanical immobilization would now be performed

- Review the fact that if a patient is standing and conscious and has no apparent major circulatory problem, no need for any immediate A B C intervention is indicated. Rather, the most urgent priority is the need to eliminate the chance of sudden collapse and its potential impact on the spine. The patient is safe from such a fall only after the backboard has been placed behind him or her and he or she is supported by the EMTs' arms under his or her armpits while grasping the board. Therefore, no delay in these steps and lowering the patient and board to the ground should occur. Once the patient has been lowered to the ground, the assessment process can continue, a rigid cervical collar can be applied, and needed treatment can begin.
- Have a participant review the immobilization of a stable standing patient to the board before it is lowered (upper torso, strap across iliac crests or groin loops, head with head immobilizer or blanket rolls, and cervical collar, NOT legs or feet)

Be sure to initial participants' Refresher Course Skill Station Summary Sheet to indicate their performance in this station, and return the sheet to them before they leave your station.

SKILL STATION 6—SPINE SKILLS "B" RAPID EXTRICATION

Purpose

The purpose of this station is to affirm and, as needed, improve the participants' ability to rapidly extricate a sitting victim from a motor vehicle directly onto a longboard while maintaining neutral spinal immobilization throughout. The intent of the station is to have the rapid extrication performed as an isolated skill *without* the need to do the initial assessment or to provide interventions during or following the extrication maneuver. The evaluator "deteriorates" the patient's condition only if too much time is spent or too much movement occurs in removing the patient.

Method

A conscious patient model is presented sitting in the driver's seat of a motor vehicle (preferably four-door sedan) and the participants are told that the vehicle struck a tree causing substantial damage to its front. The scene is safe; however the primary examination has shown that the patient's respiratory and circulatory status is compromised and unstable, requiring rapid extrication from the vehicle without delay. The team provides manual protection of the patient's spine and extricates the patient onto a longboard and away from the vehicle.

Equipment

  1 Motor vehicle (preferably four-door sedan)
  1 Patient model
  1 Longboard
  1 Rigid cervical collar properly sized to model

NOTE: Weather permitting, this station is conducted outdoors. In inclement weather it should be done under a roof (hotel overhang, parking deck, equipment bay, etc.). In extremely cold situations an enclosed place (garage, equipment bay, etc.) will be required. It should be noted that the greatest danger of exposure is to the **patient** rather than to the evaluator or participants.

The precourse planning for this station should include identifying an alternate location in the event that the weather becomes a problem on the day of the course.

Directions to Be Read to the Participants
[Introduce yourself and collect each participant's Refresher Course Skill Station Summary Sheet.]
In this station you will as a team perform a rapid extrication of a multisystem trauma patient from a motor vehicle. The scene is safe and the primary examination has been done, which reveals gross respiratory and circulatory compromise that requires immediate removal from the vehicle, stabilization, and transport. All assessment steps and interventions required before transport have already been performed. Damage to the vehicle is isolated to the front end; the doors are still functional. The patient is found sitting in the driver's seat with his back against the seat back. Do you have any questions? (Answer any).

Ask the group for the three situations in which they would perform rapid extrication instead of using a half-board or vest-type device. (Scene is unsafe, patient's medical condition is compromised and unstable, or patient blocks the EMT's access to another patient who is seriously injured)

Checklist for Use During Skill Station

- Identify the team leader and direct him or her to perform the maneuver.
- Ensures body surface isolation (BSI)
- Directs one EMT to initiate and maintain neutral, in-line immobilization of the head and neck
- Applies/directs application of cervical collar
- Positions one EMT at the front door post and another on the passenger seat
- If the EMT providing cervical immobilization is in the back seat, another EMT is positioned at the center post.
- EMT on passenger seat frees patient's legs.
- While one EMT supports the patient's thorax and another guides his or her legs, the patient is rotated in place using short moves until he has been turned 90°.
- If cervical immobilization is being provided from the back seat, the EMT performing it will be unable to completely rotate with the patient because of the center door post. At that point rotation must stop and head/neck immobilization be taken over by the EMT positioned outside the car at the center door post.
- Longboard is inserted on the seat just behind the patient.
- Patient's head and thorax are lowered to board.
- EMT at thorax places hands in patient's armpits.
- In 10 to 15 inch increments, the patient is moved along board while immobilization is maintained.
- Patient and board are moved a safe distance from vehicle (as if on cot).
- Verbalizes additional assessments/interventions that would be provided if patient's condition was reason for performing rapid extrication

- Verbalizes mechanical immobilization to longboard (straps, head immobilizer, blanket rolls, etc.)
- Verbalizes rechecking ABCs and MSC × 4.

Remediate any inadequacies or suggest changes to improve the group's performance. Have participants change roles and repeat the procedure a second time.

Be sure to initial the participants' Refresher Course Skill Station Summary Sheet to indicate their performance in this station, and return the sheet to them before they leave your station.

PART 2:
Educational Outline

Slide No.	Description	Lecture Content
R-1	*PHTLS Title Slide*	The Prehospital Trauma Life Support Course is a continuing education course developed by the Prehospital Trauma Life Support Committee of the National Association of Emergency Medical Technicians in Cooperation with the Committee on Trauma of the American College of Surgeons.
		In 1990, the PHTLS Committee identified the merit and need for a course designed distinctly as a refresher course for participants who had previously acquired the knowledge and skills included in an initial provider course.
R-2	Title Slide 2	After 2 years of development, the refresher course was completed and national dissemination was started.
		The PHTLS refresher course is designed for prehospital providers who have successfully completed a PHTLS provider course at either the basic or advanced level.
		Courses have a 3-year term of recognition. With the availability of the refresher course,

After R-2 lecture content (bulleted items):

- All PHTLS completion certificates and cards for provider and refresher courses bear an expiration date reflecting a 3-year period from course completion.
- Participants should take a refresher course at least every 3 years prior to the expiration date.

Purpose:

- The PHTLS refresher course is based upon the same content objectives and educational goals as the initial provider course you have taken.

Slide No.	Description	Lecture Content
		▪ However, because you have already acquired the knowledge and skills included, the specific objectives, the time required, and the method of presentation in the refresher course is different.

R-3	Purpose of Refresher Course
	▪ Review
	▪ Amend
	▪ Revise and Update
	▪ Reaffirm
		The PHTLS refresher course has four separate identifiable objectives:
		▪ To review the material
		  – Two, 1-hour lectures on Managing the Multisystem Trauma Patient review the key content and concepts in the provider course.
		  – Although you have had this material before, experience has shown that participants find items they have forgotten or expand their understanding of others from such a review.
		▪ To amend the original content
		  – Although the revised third edition of the text published in 1994 includes chapters on Special Considerations in Pediatric Trauma and Trauma of the Elderly, time constraints did not allow for the inclusion of all of these topics as lectures.
		  – Each topic is presented as a lecture in the refresher course.
		To revise and update
		▪ Identifying current changes in trauma care, controversies, and key items that need further study to be clearly resolved
		  – Changes in the PHTLS content, the state-of-the-art, and current literature will be identified and discussed.
		▪ Reaffirm the participants' knowledge and skills.
		  – Because individuals have both differing availability to take continuing education courses as well as differing exposure to trauma calls, it is important to reaffirm both knowledge and skill performance on the day of the course.
		  – The refresher course includes a 50-question written test that contains questions selected from each major subject area in the PHTLS course.
		  – Performing key skills in a series of skill stations will also be required. For most participants, performing the previously-learned skills to a level of competence is easily and rapidly done. Where improvement or remediation is needed, the instructors will provide it.

R-4	Trauma Summary	Conclusion summary (Faculty may choose to review items of national or regional interest in prehospital trauma management.)
R-5	Title Slide	Managing the multisystem trauma patient
R-6	Trauma	Introduction: Trauma continues to be ▪ The leading cause of death in persons 1 to 44 years of age ▪ The third leading cause of death for people of all ages in the United States ▪ The cause of death for 150,000 people each year

Slide No.	Description	Lecture Content
		▪ The American Trauma Society has estimated that at least one out of every five trauma deaths was survivable.

R-7	Causes of Trauma Deaths	▪ Trauma patients die of:
		  – A lack of adequate ventilation and oxygenation
		  – External hemorrhage
		  – Direct trauma to the thorax, abdomen, and head
		  – The fourth major cause of trauma deaths is the failure to anticipate and aggressively treat the patient for shock.

R-8	Golden Hour
	  ▪ Platinum 10 Minutes
	  ▪ Transportation
	  ▪ Emergency Department Intervention
		▪ Trauma research has shown that the key to survival for critically injured trauma patients is the initiation of definitive surgical care within 1 hour from the time of injury.
		▪ There is a decline in the number who survive for every few minutes of delay beyond this short 60-minute period known as the "Golden Hour."
		▪ Packed into the Golden Hour
		  – The time needed for dispatch and arrival at the scene
		  – The time for assessment and prehospital care to be provided at the scene
		  – The time required to transport the patient to an appropriate facility
		  – Time in the emergency department
		  – Time getting to surgery
		
		Platinum 10 Minutes
		
		▪ The EMT's main goals include being efficient, using as little of the patient's Golden Hour as possible. It is estimated that the EMT has only a "Platinum 10 Minutes" to spend with the patient at the scene. Within these few precious minutes the EMT must:
		▪ Assess the patient and recognize the critical nature of the injuries
		▪ Provide intervention only for that which is immediately lifesaving
		▪ Rapidly package the patient for transport
		▪ Any delays, any missed critical conditions, any pauses to provide care that are not truly lifesaving waste time and diminish the patient's chances for survival.
		
		Patient assessment
		
		▪ The EMT cannot treat what he or she does not find.
		  – ABCs must be evaluated quickly and properly.
		  – Even if the patient's specific problem is not readily visible, evidence of systemic danger can be found through the patient's A B C status.
		  – Based upon his or her rapid primary survey, the EMT must decide early whether the patient is a critical multisystem trauma patient or is suffering from less serious isolated trauma.
		  – If the patient is critical, the EMT must provide only immediate lifesaving care and rapidly package the patient for transport.

Slide No.	Description	Lecture Content
		– Rapidly initiated transport *is* a key *treatment* for critical trauma patients. – If the patient is not critical, the EMT continues with a full secondary assessment to find and care for all of the patient's injuries.
R-9	Priorities ▪ Scene ▪ Safety ▪ Situation	▪ The EMT's first priority on all calls must be safety of the crew and the patient. Considerations of the scene and situation come afterward. – What can these elements tell you about what has happened to the patient? ▪ Evaluate them also in terms of additional assistance that you may need: – More ambulances – Fire or rescue vehicles – Hazmat team, etc.
R-10	Automobile Crash Head-on	Determining mechanism of injury ▪ Major element of scene and situation: – What happened here? – What amount of force was involved? – Has the car windshield fractured or blown out? – Is the patient injured, fractured, or bleeding? – Is there a possibility of spinal injury? ▪ Increase the index of suspicion by evaluating the scene: – Scene – Speed – Restraints – Weapons Mechanism of injury is key indication for treatment of spinal injury ▪ Need for spinal immobilization is based on: – Mechanism of injury – Consideration of the scene, physical examination, and situation – Even if a physical examination reveals no neurologic deficit and despite the lack of positive findings, the spine should be immobilized.
R-11	Law of Conservation of Energy	▪ Law of conservation of energy – Kinetic energy (KE) is equal to one half the mass (M) times the velocity (V) squared (KE = $M/2 \times V^2$)
R-12	Blunt Trauma ▪ Shear	▪ Blunt trauma – Shear injuries were formerly referred to as "deceleration" injuries. A shear is a sudden change in movement (lateral, acceleration, deceleration, etc.) around a fixed point. – Violent squeezing forces cause compression injuries, which can produce tears and crush injuries.

Slide No.	Description	Lecture Content

R-13	Vehicular Collisions
	• Three impacts
	  – Vehicle
	  – Occupant
	  – Internal organs
		Motor vehicle injuries
		• Three impacts
		  – Vehicle
		  – Occupant
		  – Occupant's internal organs

R-14	Types of Impact
	• Head-on, frontal
	• Rear-end
	• Lateral, side
	• Rotational, pivot
	• Roll-over
		• Direction and type of impact has a major role in determining type and extent of possible injuries.
		• Lateral impacts
		• Lateral impact with flail chest and impaled femur noted
		• Lateral impacts produce unusual results that are worth reviewing:
		  – Thorax: lateral rib fractures, lateral flail segment, pulmonary contusions, or aortic tears. Liver and spleen injuries occur from lateral rather than frontal impact.
		  – Lateral impact at hip forces head of femur laterally into the acetabulum. Pelvic fractures may be present.
		  – C-spine is damaged as head moves laterally.
		  – Occupant's head impacts on head or shoulder of other passenger or on interior side wall of car, resulting in contusions and hemorrhage.
		  – Be alert to injuries caused to patient's side by seat belt harness (driver's right, passenger's left).
		  – Lesson to be learned: when the impact is from the side, the injuries will most likely also be on the side.
		• Drag destruction: bullet traveling through body, with tumble and yaw
		• Penetrating injuries
		  – The greater the speed of the bullet, the greater its injury potential. When a bullet enters the body and exits, it creates tissue damage equal to the amount of speed it lost while traveling through the body. The entrance velocity minus the exit velocity equals the kinetic energy (KE) of the damage. When there is no exit wound, all of the bullet's kinetic energy is transformed into bodily damage.
		  – Bullets present an additional consideration. The profile of the bullet adds an extra dimension to the damage that it can cause. "Mushrooming," or fragmenting or tumbling, upon impact causes additional slowing—and the amount of resulting tissue damage is directly related to the reduction in speed of the bullet as it passes through the body. Bullet design can be more damaging than size. Bullets which are designed for hunting (to kill) are more damaging than bullets designed to maim or stop.
		• Area of possible damage: Knife stab wound showing blade and internal cone of damage
		• Pathway—Stab wound
		  – A small entrance wound does not indicate a small amount of damage because blade may have moved through a larger (cone-shaped) area once inside the body.
		  – An associated injury must be suspected and may include any structures and organs that were within the length and potential articulation of the penetrating object.

Slide No.	Description	Lecture Content

- Zones of damage: Internal damage cavity: (L) medium energy, (R) high energy
- Cavitation
  - More velocity, more damage
  - Passage of bullet produces path of absolute tissue damage that is related to size of bullet
  - Greater damage is caused by cavitation. The speed (motion energy) of the bullet causes a cavity to form as the "shock wave" drives tissue away from the bullet's path. The new temporary cavity is much larger than the damage caused by the bullet itself.
  - The energy causes tissue damage equal to the bullet's amount of motion energy.
- Global survey:
  - Provides a quick overview of the patient's overall condition
  - Is a simultaneous evaluation of the patient's airway, breathing, circulation, and gross levels of consciousness, including visual clues of external hemorrhage
  - Includes considerations of scene, situation, and mechanism of injury and takes only a few seconds to accomplish
  - The EMT's next step is to perform the rest of the primary survey.

R-15

Primary Survey
- Global assessment
- In-depth systems
- Locate life-threatening injuries
- Manage life-threatening conditions found

The goal of the primary survey is to locate all critical injuries and any life-threatening conditions such as shock.

- The primary survey is performed in sequence by checking the:
  - Airway
  - Breathing
  - Circulation
  - Gross neurologic status, by exposing the body as needed to evaluate an injury
- During the primary survey, critical problems are managed when they are found. There is nothing to be gained by continuing the survey until these problems are corrected.

R-16

Airway Management
- Manual
- Mechanical

Airway management

- The first step is to assess and manage the airway as needed and maintain in-line cervical support. EMTs must be aggressive in their approach to the airway.
- Manual airway methods
  - Trauma chin lift
  - Trauma jaw thrust
- Mechanical methods
  - Oral and nasal airways are mechanical devices that can be used with C-spine measures to help maintain a patent airway. Nasopharyngeal airways can be used on patients who still have a gag reflex.
  - The preferred method of airway management in critical patients is endotracheal intubation performed with C-spine immobilization techniques.

Slide No.	Description	Lecture Content
R-17	Ventilation Minute Volume	▪ The second step in the primary survey is breathing. – Is the patient breathing? – Adequate air exchange? – Auscultate to be sure that air is actually moving through the lungs. – The key to assessing breathing is to determine the minute volume. "MV" is the volume of air which passes into and out of the lungs each minute—the ventilatory rate multiplied by the tidal volume. – When the breathing rate is too slow, it will not move enough oxygen each minute to adequately perfuse the cells. If the breathing rate is too fast, there will not be enough volume with each breath to provide adequate perfusion.
R-18	Ventilatory Rate	▪ Suspect ventilatory compromise in any patient who is breathing less than 12 or more than 20 times per minute. Be ready to aggressively assist ventilation if any other signs of respiratory compromise or deficit are found. – Expect to manage the breathing of any patient who is breathing less than 10 or more than 30 times per minute. Be ready to provide assisted breathing with a bag-valve-mask device, complete with oxygen supply and reservoir. – Treat aggressively—the patient's life depends on it!
R-19	Oxygen Concentrations	▪ Patients need adequate oxygen. – The concentration of oxygen delivered depends on the liter flow rate and the equipment used. – A nasal cannula is not recommended for the critical trauma patient; the concentration delivered is below 50% and is inadequate. – If the patient is breathing adequately, a non-rebreather reservoir mask should be used. – If a bag-valve-mask device is used, it must be connected to oxygen and a reservoir to provide concentrations of 85% to 95%.
R-20	Goal: Ensure Adequate Oxygenation of Cells ▪ Manage airway ▪ Ensure adequate ventilation ▪ Ensure adequate oxygenation	▪ Assessing breathing also means looking for any physical problem which could inhibit ventilation, such as injury to the neck or thorax. – Examine the chest thoroughly for problems that interfere with the ability to breathe. – Airway and ventilatory deficits are the causes of death in trauma patients. – Expect every trauma patient to have a compromised airway and ventilation until proven otherwise.
R-21	Circulation ▪ Pulse ▪ Skin ▪ Capillary refill	Circulation ▪ Assess circulation by checking: – Pulse presence and rate – Skin color, moisture, and temperature

Slide No.	Description	Lecture Content
	■ Overt hemorrhage ■ Consider shock	– Capillary refill – For any signs of gross external hemorrhage ■ Consider the whole patient when evaluating for the potential of shock.
R-22	Adequate Circulation ■ Pump ■ Volume of fluid ■ Container	■ Adequate circulation of blood depends upon three main factors: – A pump that can effectively move blood through the vascular system – A container, or closed system of blood vessels to carry the blood – An adequate volume of blood to fill the system ■ Each of these elements is dependent upon the others. If the container becomes too large for the amount of blood in the system, or if the amount of blood decreases and the container size stays the same, the pump's effectiveness will diminish.
R-23	Fick Principle ■ Adequately oxygenated RBCs ■ Adequate number of RBCs ■ Adequate circulation of oxygenated RBCs ■ RBCs able to off-load oxygen to cells	Shock ■ Cellular oxygenation is the movement of oxygen from the alveoli to cells throughout the body. It involves four main steps: – Red blood cells (RBCs) able to receive or "on-load" oxygen from the alveolar capillaries – There must be enough RBCs – The circulatory system must be able to move the oxygenated RBCs throughout the body – The body's biochemical balance must allow the oxygen to be "off-loaded" from the RBCs through the cellular membranes and into the cells ■ When all of these elements are present, the body functions in aerobic (oxygen-based) metabolism at the cellular level. The alternative is shock.
R-24	Cellular Response to Shock ■ Anaerobic metabolism ■ Cellular death ■ Organ death ■ Organism death	■ Cellular response to shock ■ Systemic hypoperfusion of cells causing cellular hypoxia results in the inability of the cells to receive and use amounts of oxygen for fuel. – Poor cardiac output from a failure in either the pump, the container, or the volume of blood causes hypotension. – This leads to hypoperfusion of the cells, cellular hypoxia, and anaerobic metabolism. – When anaerobic metabolism occurs for long enough, the cells die. – As cells die, so do the organs made up of those cells. When enough organs die, or when an organ essential to life dies, the organism dies.
R-25	Management of Shock in the *First Hour* Determines Outcome 2 to 21 Days Later	■ The progression from cellular death to organism death is not immediate. – It is a quiet process that can begin in the first minutes after an injury and may take 2, 10, or even 21 days to conclude with the patient's death.

Slide No.	Description	Lecture Content

- The EMT's actions to support circulation and reverse the outward signs of shock are geared to keeping the patient alive days later.
- When the EMT fails to treat for shock, he or she is contributing to the patient's eventual death just as much as, if not more than, the patient's injuries.

Shock assessment summary

- Shock develops in stages that are identified by outward signs and symptoms.
  - "Compensated" shock occurs first. The body's normal defense mechanisms work to overcome the developing hypotension and hypoperfusion.
  - "Uncompensated" shock is the second stage, when the defense mechanisms are unable to compensate for the systemic decline caused by poor circulation.
  - "Irreversible" shock is a terminal event—the body has been unable to overcome the effects of anaerobic metabolism and the death of vital organs.
  - Early signs of shock, indicative of the compensatory stage, include:
    - Tachycardia
    - Changes in skin color, moisture, and temperature
  - In compensated shock, changes are seen in:
    - Blood pressure
    - Level of consciousness
    - Pulse rate and skin
- The patient's survival depends directly on the EMT's ability to provide aggressive and appropriate circulatory resuscitation.

R-26 Neurologic Assessment
- Check responsiveness
- Check pupils
- Check for deficit

- Neurologic assessment
- The neurologic assessment in the primary survey is limited to a gross check for level of responsiveness, pupillary reaction, and motor deficit.
  - The "AVPU" index is helpful in determining if the patient is alert and oriented, responsive to verbal stimulus, responsive only to painful stimulus, or completely unresponsive.
  - Pupils should be quickly checked for equal size and reactivity.
  - Motor ability, sensory response, and circulation should be quickly checked in all four extremities (MSC × 4) to identify localized problems as well as superior-to-inferior and left-to-right motor deficits.
  - A more complete neurologic assessment is done in the secondary survey if time permits. This "quick-look" tells the EMT if there are major brain or nervous system problems to consider and may also reveal other systemic problems that are presenting as neurologic signs and symptoms.

Expose, examine, evaluate

- A final stop in the primary survey is to expose, examine, and evaluate any areas of the body in which a serious condition or injury has been found or of which the EMT has been unable to directly observe.

Slide No.	Description	Lecture Content

– If it has not been done already, this is also the time to quickly check the abdomen for distension or gross tenderness that may indicate an intra-abdominal injury.

R-27 | **Keys to Effective Prehospital Care**
- Early recognition
- Meaningful intervention
- Efficiency of care
- Rapid intervention

- Shock management
- Efficiency is one of the keys to appropriate management of the critical trauma patient.
  – Recognize the nature of injuries quickly and transport.
  – Be organized and efficient in delivering lifesaving care that the patient needs.
    – IVs take time to set up and start even in the best of conditions. Time spent at the scene to start an IV wastes the patient's Platinum 10 Minutes. IVs are usually best started during transport.

R-28 | **Management: Shock**

- Prehospital management of shock from trauma begins with aggressive management of airway, breathing, and circulation. The key elements in treating shock are:
  – Positioning the patient supine on a long backboard
  – Retaining the patient's natural body heat to avoid vasodilation as a response to being cold
  – High FiO_2 oxygen enrichment
  – Pneumatic antishock garment inflated at the scene as indicated
  – Two IVs of Ringer's lactate—with large bore catheters and tubing started while en route
  – Rapidly initiating transport to the nearest appropriate hospital

R-29 | **Resuscitation Phase**
- Correct key problems as found
- Reevaluate

Resuscitation phase
Key problems should be found and corrected during the primary survey

- After the primary survey the EMT should pause to evaluate all of his or her findings.
  – Are any additional resuscitation measures called for?
  – Should any treatment that is already in place be changed or upgraded? For example, if bag-valve-mask ventilation is underway, should intubation now be done?

Evaluate patient's condition.

- Now evaluate the patient's overall status and determine if this is:
  – A multisystem trauma patient
  – A case of simple, isolated trauma
  – Mentally review the patient's signs and symptoms.
    – Are they consistent or is there evidence of a systemic problem that is not explained by the injuries that have been found?
    – Is the patient hypoxic or in shock?
    – Have all other etiologies been ruled out?
- If the primary survey reveals only simple, isolated trauma, the secondary survey should be done before moving the patient.
- If the patient is a multisystem trauma patient, the EMT must forego any further assessment at the scene and focus on providing only lifesaving resuscitative measures.

Slide No.	Description	Lecture Content

– Rapid packaging
– Immediately initiate transport to an appropriate facility.
– Secondary assessment can be done en route if time permits.

Rapid extrication and multisystem trauma

- Every multisystem trauma patient must be assumed to have a compromised spine in addition to any other injuries. Usual spine techniques can take 6 to 10 minutes to perform. Learn and utilize such methods as rapid extrication to manually immobilize the spine while moving the patient directly onto a long backboard.

Definitive field care: Simple isolated trauma

- If the patient is suffering only from simple, isolated trauma, the EMT's prehospital care consists of:
  – Ruling out the possibility of multisystem traumas. This cannot be overstated. The EMT must remain suspicious that the patient is more injured than has been so far discovered and must continually recheck and reevaluate for signs of shock or systemic involvement.
  – Performing a complete secondary survey
  – Bandaging all open wounds, stabilizing all fractures, and appropriately packaging the patient for transport
  – Providing careful appropriate transportation

Definitive field care: Multisystem trauma

- The critical patient needs lifesaving care and immediate transport to a facility that can provide the blood and surgical intervention to keep him or her alive.
  – Rapid packaging on a longboard supports, protects, and immobilizes all parts of the body in one quick efficient step.
  – If the EMT responds inappropriately and treats the critical patient for every minor injury, the chances for survival will be greatly reduced.

Slide No.	Description	Lecture Content
R-30	Title Slide	Managing the multisystem trauma patient
R-31	Thoracic Trauma Deaths • Inadequate ventilation • Inadequate circulation	Specific injuries—thorax Thoracic injuries can produce a particularly rapid deterioration in the patient's condition. Trauma patients are vulnerable to a deadly sequence of events if the ventilatory or circulatory systems are compromised.

- Inadequate ventilation results in low oxygen levels in the alveoli.
- Inadequate circulation results in hypoperfusion.
- Both are final stops in the development of systemic hypoxia and shock.
- The principal ways in which this circulorespiratory compromise can occur include changes in:
  – Chest wall motion
  – Lung expansion
  – Oxygen diffusion in the capillaries
  – Circulation

Slide No.	Description	Lecture Content
R-32	Pathophysiology • Changes in chest wall motion • Changes in lung expansion • Changes in diffusion • Changes in circulation	Thoracic trauma can inhibit adequate ventilation by restricting the amount of oxygen that can move in and out of the lungs. • This results from a loss of integrity of the chest wall, such as with a flail chest or a sucking wound where there is a direct opening to the outside. • Less common is neurologic damage which prevents the intercostal muscles from expanding the thoracic cage. • This category also includes cases where chest wall motion is restricted by external force that prevents the chest wall from moving, such as cave-ins and building collapses. Even if the chest wall is intact and able to move freely, any condition which restricts lung expansion and relaxation will result in inadequate alveolar oxygenation. • The majority of conditions which affect lung expansion are directly associated with thoracic trauma: – Closed pneumothorax – Tension pneumothorax – Open pneumothorax – Hemothorax • Extreme abdominal distention can cause the diaphragm to bulge upward, exerting increased intrathoracic pressure on the lungs. Some conditions can affect the diffusion of oxygen and other gases across the alveolar membrane. Even though oxygen is present in the lungs it is unable to reach the circulating hemoglobin, and cellular hypoxia results. These can include: • Pulmonary contusions • Pulmonary edema • Chemical imbalances which limit the transfer of oxygen across the cell membrane. Changes in circulation can result in critical thoracic problems. Although each condition is different, the net result is a decrease in the circulation of oxygenated RBCs due to a compromise in the thorax. These include: • Blood loss into the thorax • Pericardial tamponade • Myocardial contusion • Tension pneumothorax • A decrease in the amount of blood returning to the heart due to hemorrhage elsewhere in the body
R-33	Rib Fractures • Single isolated rib fractures • Multiple fractures may produce "flail chest"	Among the chest injuries which the EMT may encounter are single isolated rib fractures and multiple fractures of adjacent ribs. • Simple fractures by themselves do not present a true emergency unless the pain associated with inspiration is so great that it prevents adequate breathing. • Multiple fractures that result in a flail chest do present a true emergency. – The pulmonary contusion associated with a flail segment prevents adequate respiration and leads to a rapid deterioration of the patient into hypoxia and shock. – Paradoxical movement of the chest wall resulting from a flail segment inhibits adequate ventilation and leads to hypoxia and shock.

Slide No.	Description	Lecture Content
		• The flail chest patient should be ventilated with a high FiO_2 using a positive pressure device.
		• The flail segment can be stabilized by taping or strapping, although this is less important than adequate ventilation and oxygenation.
		• The use of sandbags to stabilize a flail chest is contraindicated; the excessive weight further inhibits the patient's ventilation. Similarly, the use of tape or bandages which fully encircle the thorax is also not recommended; this limits chest excursion and further inhibits ventilation.
R-34	Title Slide	Closed pneumothorax
R-35	Closed Pneumothorax	Closed pneumothorax

• Frequently not an emergency
• The EMT should provide only such supportive treatment as may be required.
• The real concern is that it may progress undetected into a tension pneumothorax.
• The importance of a simple pneumothorax also varies according to the skill level of the responding EMT.
  – For an EMT-paramedic who has been trained and certified to perform needle decompression, the consequences of a simple pneumothorax progressing to tension are not as catastrophic as for a basic or advanced level EMT.
  – When the EMTs caring for a patient with a simple pneumothorax are unable to decompress a chest, the level of urgency in reaching an appropriate medical facility increases.

Paper-bag syndrome

The "paper-bag syndrome" describes a mechanism of chest injury which is a leading cause of pneumothorax.

• Patients who anticipate a violent collision instinctively trap air in their lungs.
• The hyperinflated lungs become an additional hazard to the patient when the chest wall is suddenly compressed by the steering wheel or dashboard in a frontal collision.
• The compressive forces, coupled with the extra air trapped in the lungs, can result in a ruptured lung, trachea-bronchial tears, and increased chances of pulmonary contusion.

Open pneumothorax

An open pneumothorax, resulting in a "sucking chest wound," is a true emergency which requires rapid recognition and intervention.

• Wound should be closed with an occlusive dressing
• The patient should be given high FiO_2 and ventilated with positive pressure if required.

Tension pneumothorax

A tension pneumothorax may develop from a closed pneumothorax or from an open pneumothorax which has been sealed by the EMT.

• As air passes from the bronchi through the hole in the lung and into the pleural space, the pressure inside that half of the thorax increases and begins to press upon the uninjured lung and other thoracic organs.

- The heart's ability to pump can be compromised by pressure on the heart itself or by decreased cardiac return.
- LATE signs of tension pneumothorax are mediastinal shift and tracheal deviation.
- A tension pneumothorax is a true life-threatening emergency.

Occlusive dressing being resealed over chest wound

- If the patient has an open chest wound which was sealed by the EMT, a corner of the occlusive dressing should be opened to release the pressure.
- A sudden marked improvement should be seen.
- The dressing can then be reapplied and patient monitoring continued.
- If the tension pneumothorax is not associated with an open chest wound, the EMT must:
  - Perform a needle decompression of the chest (if properly trained and certified), **or**
  - Provide immediate rapid transportation to the closest appropriate facility.

Hemothorax

A hemothorax may develop from one of several causes and frequently presents as a combination hemopneumothorax, with both air and blood in the pleural space.

- The presence of blood inside the thorax decreases the space available for lung expansion and can inhibit myocardial motion in extreme cases.
- The more common and greater problem is the loss of circulating blood volume.
  - A patient can lose more than a liter of blood into each side of the thorax before signs of dyspnea or muffled breath sounds become apparent.
  - Primary treatment should be for hypovolemic shock.
  - The use of the PASG in such patients is often not indicated because conventional hypovolemic shock therapy will cause increased bleeding in the patient's thorax. The EMT should communicate with medical control for direction.

Torn aorta

Aortic tears are the classic "shear" or "deceleration" injuries.

- Survival statistics on patients with aortic tears are abysmally low, and little improvement can be expected if EMTs do not become more alert and responsive to this condition.
- If the aorta has been opened at the time of injury, the EMT will invariably find a pulseless patient when he or she arrives at the scene.
- At times, however, the aorta has only been damaged and a traumatic aneurysm develops—a time bomb waiting to rupture.
- The EMT's suspicion and report of the situation and mechanism of injury are key in alerting the receiving emergency department staff to the problem.

Slide No.	Description	Lecture Content

Myocardial contusion
    Myocardial contusions result in damage to heart muscle tissue.

- Chest wall bruising is usually, but not always, seen.
- Fractured ribs or other more overt chest trauma may or may not be present.
- The EMT's level of suspicion and evaluation of the scene and situation are key.
- A myocardial contusion compromises circulation.
    - The heart cannot pump effectively because of damaged muscle tissue.
    - Cardiac monitor may display dysrhythmias indicative of the damage.
- EMT must balance treating a trauma patient who also has cardiac problems.
    - ACLS protocols can be followed in treating the dysrhythmias.
    - This is also a trauma patient whose other injuries can be equally lethal.

R-36 — Pericardial Tamponade
- Pathophysiology

Pericardial tamponade

- No visible external signs may be present.
- As blood fills the pericardial sac, pressure is exerted on the ventricles and restricts their ability to fill between compressions.
- This causes reduced stroke volume, which decreases cardiac output and reduces circulation of oxygenated red blood cells throughout the body.
- No specific prehospital care is possible except suspicion and recognition, communication with the receiving staff, rapid transport to an appropriate facility, and general symptomatic support.

R-37 — Thoracic Trauma
- Management

The management of thoracic trauma is based on the key concepts of:

- Restoring adequate ventilation
- Providing high FiO_2 ventilation
- Closing open chest wall wounds
- Stabilizing fractures
- Relieving tension pneumothorax when present
- Rapidly initiating transport to an appropriate facility

R-38 — Abdominal Trauma
- Pathophysiology
- Key indicator

Specific injuries—Abdomen
Abdominal trauma usually presents as a problem of either injury hemorrhage and/or the spilling of caustic matter from various organs into the abdomen.

- Key signs and symptoms:
    - History and mechanism of injury
    - Visible external bruising
    - Distention of the abdomen
    - Pain or tenderness on palpation
- The presence of palpable or pulsatile masses is also significant, but these signs take time to develop and they may be absent during the initial assessment.

Slide No.	Description	Lecture Content

Lap belt versus internal organs

Blunt trauma can result in damaged organs and torn blood vessels. In this illustration an IMPROPERLY worn lap belt serves as a rigid barrier as the body moves forward, compressing the abdominal organs between the posterior abdominal wall and spinal column and the belt.

Diaphragmatic herniation

The diaphragm can herniate from increased abdominal pressure.

- Pushes abdominal organs into the thorax
- Reduces volume of thorax
- Combined thoracic-abdominal problem
- Can also occur when penetrating wounds puncture the diaphragm
- Can create a sucking abdominal wound.

Liver moving against ligamentum teres

Abdominal organs can also be injured by "shear" or "deceleration" injuries

- The momentum of internal organs against bones and ligaments can produce significant injuries.
- Classic example: liver moving forward against the ligamentum teres.

R-39

Suspect Intra-abdominal Bleeding

- When signs of shock are NOT explained by other serious injuries
  – Head injury
  – Thoracic injury
  – External hemorrhage

Intra-abdominal bleeding may occur without open wounds, and signs may not be immediately present.

- Suspect intra-abdominal bleeding whenever the patient's level of shock cannot be explained by other serious injuries.
  – Bleeding into the head presents decreasing levels of consciousness and specific neurologic signs.
  – More than a liter of blood in the thorax causes increasing dyspnea and decreased unilateral breath sounds.
  – External hemorrhage is evidenced by the presence of blood and external wounds.
- If the patient is in shock but none of these other injury patterns are present, the EMT should suspect the patient of having an intra-abdominal bleed and should treat accordingly.

R-40

"On Scene" Management

The prehospital management of abdominal trauma can be broken into two phases:

- "On scene" priorities are:
  – Ventilation as needed
  – Hemorrhage control, usually involving the pneumatic anti-shock garment
  – Rapidly packaging the patient for immediate transport to a facility where surgical care is readily available
- Survival time of patients with serious abdominal trauma is directly linked to the time span from injury to definitive hemorrhage control.

Slide No.	Description	Lecture Content

R-41	"En route" Management	"En route" priorities expand to:
		▪ High FiO$_2$ ventilation
		▪ Treat for shock:
		  – Continue PASG
		  – Maintain body temperature
		  – Start IVs
		  – The patient's needs center around definitive control of hemorrhage and replacing lost blood. Neither can be done in the field.
		▪ Abdominal eviscerations
		  – Do not become distracted by the gross appearance of any abdominal wounds.
		  – Cover eviscerations with large, moist dressings.
		  – Follow the general rules of care for abdominal injuries.
		  – Inflate only the leg compartments of the PASG unless the patient cannot be stabilized or begins to deteriorate.
		  – Contact medical control for physician directions.

R-42	Head Trauma: Pathophysiology	Specific injuries—Head
		Head injuries and resulting respiratory compromise represents the single largest cause of trauma deaths.
		▪ Head injuries include:
		  – Scale hemorrhage
		  – Skull fractures
		  – Concussions and contusions
		  – Intracranial hemorrhage
		  – Direct massive brain damage
		▪ The signs and symptoms of head trauma include:
		  – Changes in level of consciousness
		  – Motor and/or sensory deficits between the right and left sides
		  – Changes in ventilatory pattern
		  – Convulsions
		  – Focal motor signs
		  – Unusual behavior such as combativeness and inappropriate responses to verbal or painful stimuli

R-43	Head Trauma
	▪ Skull Fractures
	  – Depressed
	  – Linear
	▪ Basilar Fractures
	  – CSF from ears, nose
	  – Bleeding from ears
	  – Raccoon Eyes
	  – Battle's Sign
		Skull fractures
		▪ Signs:
		  – Cerebrospinal fluid (CSF) leaking from the ears, nose, or mouth
		  – Any bleeding from within the ear or nose
		  – Great significance when assessing for head injury
		  – When CSF is associated with blood, it produces a bulls-eye pattern when dripped onto a towel or piece of paper.
		▪ Two other signs may appear relatively late. Their absence is not a reliable "rule out" of a basilar skull fracture:
		  – Periorbital ecchymosis, or "Raccoon Eyes"
		  – Ecchymosis behind the ears, or "Battle's Sign"
		  – If either is present, the fracture may be several hours old or the condition may have progressed further than first suspected.

Slide No.	Description	Lecture Content

Head strike with examples of injuries

Any flow of CSF or blood from the ears, nose, or mouth indicates an OPEN skull fracture.

- Do NOT try to stop the flow, as a blockage can cause increased intracranial pressure.
- Do not place localized direct pressure over any open or depressed skull fracture to avoid pushing bone shards into the brain tissue.
- If scalp bleeding is profuse, a wide-area pressure dressing can be used. Dressings should be placed over open skull fractures to help avoid infection.
- The presence of an open or depressed skull fracture is a dire emergency.
  - Keep the head elevated if possible.
  - Provide symptomatic support treatment.
  - Rapidly initiate transport to facility.

R-44 | Concussion and Contusion

The two most common types of closed head injuries are concussions and contusions.

- Concussions are a "shaking up" of the brain without the skull.
  - Characterized by a loss of consciousness which lasts less than 5 minutes.
  - No permanent injury or deficit results from a concussion.
- A contusion is a more significant injury.
  - Bruising of the brain
  - Development of occhymosis
  - Loss of consciousness greater than 5 minutes
  - Focal neurologic changes
  - Patient may suffer some lasting neurologic deficit.
- Prehospital care for both conditions is symptomatic support, oxygen, and rapidly initiated transport to an appropriate medical facility.

Intracranial anatomy

To better understand intracranial bleeding, it is necessary to review the cranial anatomy.

- Outermost layer is the scalp: comprises skin, hair follicles, and various blood vessels and nerves
- Beneath the scalp is the rigid bony skull, or cranium
- Beneath the skull and above the dura mater is the epidural space, a "potential" space in which the meningeal arteries are found and into which bleeding can occur.
- The dura mater is a tough, inelastic covering beneath the skull and above the brain.
- Below the dura mater is a spiderlike membrane called the arachnoid and below it is the pia mater, which is the covering of the brain itself.
- The pia mater and arachnoid do not touch at every point, and the area between the two is called the subarachnoid space and contains meningeal veins and cerebrospinal fluid.

Slide No.	Description	Lecture Content
R-45	Intracranial Hemorrhage	Intracranial hemorrhage—bleeding inside the cranium—falls into three categories:
		▪ Epidural, or above the dura mater – Originates from the meningeal arteries and occurs in the potential space between the cranium and the dura mater – High incidence of fatality – Must be immediately recognized and treated surgically if the patient is to survive ▪ Subdural, occurring below the dura in the subdural space or between layers of the dura mater—not in the brain itself ▪ Intracerebral, or in the brain itself – Can be a devastatingly rapid cause of death – The signs and symptoms of the various types of intracranial bleeding vary depending on both the specific location of the hemorrhage and also the amount of increased intracranial pressure caused by the bleeding.
R-46	Subdural Hematomas ▪ Acute ▪ Subacute ▪ Chronic	Subdural hematomas are classified as acute, subacute, or chronic. ▪ Acute present in the first 24 hours after injury ▪ Subacute display more slowly, usually in 25 to 64 hours. ▪ Chronic may develop weeks or even months after the injury and may be caused by an otherwise seemingly minor head injury.
R-47	Suspect Possible Subdural Hematoma	The EMT should suspect a possible subdural hematoma if called days, weeks, or even months after a head injury and when any of the following signs or symptoms are displayed: ▪ Nausea or vomiting ▪ Persistent or recurring headache ▪ Changes in vision ▪ Somnolence ▪ Personality changes or inappropriate behavior ▪ Changes in mentation or fine motor skills ▪ One-sided paralysis, weakness, or loss of feeling ▪ Changes in level of consciousness: confusion or disorientation, coma
R-48	Head Trauma: Physiology ▪ Cerebral perfusion ▪ Mean arterial pressure	Cerebral perfusion pressure (CPP) ▪ Difference between mean arterial pressure (MAP) and intracranial pressure (ICP). ▪ When MAP falls or ICP rises, brain perfusion diminishes. ▪ When ICP increases, cerebral blood vessels are compressed and the flow of blood to the brain decreases. ▪ Cerebral arterial response tries to overcome the decreased perfusion by directly activating the sympathetic nervous system. The release of catecholamines results in an increased blood pressure. ▪ Normally, stimulating the sympathetic system would also increase heart rate; however, the pulse does not increase in these cases because the increased ICP also stimulates the vagus nerve.

Slide No.	Description	Lecture Content
R-49	CO_2 is a Potent Vasodilator • Increased intracranial pressure	Carbon dioxide (CO_2) is a potent vasodilator • When the level of CO_2 in the arteries ($PaCO_2$) rises above the normal range, it causes the blood vessels to dilate. – This increases the amount of space that the blood vessels take up in the skull, which in turn . . . – Causes a rise in intracranial pressure – And restricts the flow of oxygenated blood to the brain cells – The resulting cerebral hypoxia produces edema in the brain, adding further to the problem of increased intracranial pressure. • By contrast, when the patient is hyperoxygenated, the PaO_2 rises and cerebral edema is reduced.
R-50	CO_2 is a Potent Vasodilator • Hyperventilation • Hyperoxygenation	• Hyperventilation allows CO_2 to be "blown off". – As the $PaCO_2$ returns to normal level, vasoconstriction occurs. – The vascular volume inside the skull decreases. – The intracranial pressure lowers. – 24 to 30 breaths per minute
R-51	Spine and Musculoskeletal Trauma • Pathophysiology	Trauma to the spine does not commonly cause death; however, it can result in lifelong paralysis. Injuries can include: • Vertebral fractures • Displacement or subluxation of vertebrae • Overstretching of the muscles and ligaments attached to the spinal column. The spinal column may be injured or rendered unstable without any damage occurring to the spinal cord. • Patient with a damaged spinal column may present without cord symptoms. • EMT's attitude must be that the cord has not yet been injured. • EMT must do everything possible to protect the cord. When the cord is damaged, the EMT sees symptoms consistent with neurologic changes and motorsensory deficits.
R-52	Spine Trauma • A lack of neurologic deficit does not rule out an unstable spine.	A lack of neurologic deficit does not rule out the possibility of an unstable spinal column—it indicates only that no spinal cord damage has as yet occurred. It does not rule out musculoskeletal damage or instability. Restrained driver presents with head that can still move forward. Mechanism of injury • Key indication that the patient requires spinal immobilization, regardless of negative findings or the absence of symptoms • Even when fully restrained in a motor vehicle collision, the potential for spinal trauma is not eliminated. • The combination of lap and shoulder belts protect the abdomen, chest, face, and head from impacting with the vehicle's interior; however, the head continues to move forward, causing sudden and extreme hyperflexion and a potentially unstable spine.

Slide No.	Description	Lecture Content

■ Any sudden violent lateral movement, such as that produced by a car being struck from the side, can also create serious spine trauma even in a restrained victim.

R-53

Spine Trauma
■ Signs
■ Symptoms

Signs and symptoms

■ Consider the presence of other injuries indicative of sudden violent force to any part of the spine.
  – Massive trauma to the head, face, or chest
  – Broken helmet
  – Any head injury with changes in level of consciousness
  – Bulls-eye windshield fracture
  – Lateral injuries to the pelvis
■ Other important signs and symptoms include:
  – Pain, with or without movement
  – Pain on palpation
  – Deformity or guarding
  – Paralysis, weakness, numbness, tingling, or motor deficit
  – Any sign of vasodilation associated with neurologic shock
  – Priapism in males

Skeleton and boarded patient in parallel postures

Management

■ Immobilization in a neutral, in-line position supine on a long backboard
■ Immobilization is like pregnancy—either you are or you aren't; there is no "almost" or "partial" degree of immobilization. An all too common error made by EMTs is the failure to properly immobilize spine-injured patients.
■ The goal is to immobilize spine patients so that they cannot move up, down, or to either side.

R-54

Spine Trauma
Summary
■ Method

Principles of management

■ Provide manual, in-line support of the head and neck
■ Evaluate
  – ABCs
  – Need for immediate resuscitation
  – Situation in general; is there a need for immediate removal (rapid extrication)?
■ Apply a properly fitting cervical collar.
■ Check motor, sensory and circulatory functions in all four extremities (MSC × 4)
■ Apply an interim spinal immobilization device if the patient cannot be moved directly to a longboard.
■ Move the patient and device to the longboard and secure both to the board. Strap the patient's legs to the board and tie the feet together. These last two steps complete the immobilization process by preventing movement of the feet and legs, which could twist or move the pelvis and thereby affect the spine.
■ Recheck ABCs and MSC × 4

Slide No.	Description	Lecture Content
R-55	Musculoskeletal Trauma • Priorities of care • Missed injuries	Specific injuries—extremity Frequently considered "forgotten" trauma because higher priority has been placed on head, chest, and abdominal injuries. Extremity trauma can also be life threatening: • Severe external hemorrhage • Concealed internal hemorrhage These must be included in the primary survey along with all A B C life-threatening injuries. In the multisystem trauma patient: • It is NOT appropriate for the EMT to splint and bandage every fracture or extremity injury. • It is NOT appropriate for the EMT to overlook life-threatening extremity injuries in any patient or to carelessly miss extremity trauma in patients with only minor injuries.
R-56	All Musculoskeletal Injuries Must be Treated as Fractures by EMTs	Wide range of possible extremity injuries: • Fractures • Dislocations • Sprains • Strains • Combinations of each of these • EMT must treat all as possible fractures until the patient can be X-rayed and evaluated by a physician.
R-57	Musculoskeletal Trauma: Special Considerations • Concealed internal bleeding	Concealed internal bleeding • Any long-bone fracture can produce 500 to 1500 ml of blood. • A femur fracture can produce up to 1500 ml of concealed bleeding in each thigh. • A fractured pelvis can allow even greater amounts of blood loss. • Traction splints and the PASG can aid in controlling internal hemorrhage by reducing the amount of any "third space" capsule which may have been created by overriding bone ends.
R-58	Title Slide—Thermal Injuries	
R-59	Burn Trauma • Immediate measures to save lives	Specific injuries—burns Key considerations: • Safety of EMT and patient • Stop the burning. The patient does not benefit if carelessness causes the EMT to be injured or killed when responding to the scene.
R-60	First Treat Other Trauma, then Treat the Burn!	Burn patients are TRAUMA patients first and burn patients SECOND. The EMT should focus his or her priorities just as for any trauma patient: • Treat any life-threatening conditions found. • Then treat the burn.

Slide No.	Description	Lecture Content
		Most burn patients who die in the first few hours die from airway and breathing problems. ■ The EMT must aggressively focus on opening and controlling the airway, providing high flow percentage oxygen, and assisting ventilation. ■ Shock, if seen early in the burn patient, is rarely caused by the burn but rather by other injuries. ■ The EMT must check for other life-threatening injuries, especially those that may be accompanied by external or internal hemorrhage, and must consider the possibility of carbon monoxide poisoning or the influence of other noxious gasses. ■ Pain contributes to the development of shock.
R-61	Burn Trauma ■ Smoke inhalation	Special complications: smoke inhalation ■ Inhalation of smoke and noxious fumes can jeopardize the patient's airway through inflammation and edema. ■ In severe cases, it can cause sloughing of the tracheobronchial tree. ■ The severity of inhalation injuries is determined by: – Toxicity of the product – Concentration or density – Amount inhaled – Duration of exposure ■ Whenever a burn patient has been in an enclosed space, carbon monoxide poisoning must be considered as a possible risk, and transportation to the hospital is required.
R-62	Chemical Burns ■ Management ■ Remove the agent	Special complications: chemical burns ■ Remove all traces of the substance from the patient in order to stop the burning process: – Dilute liquids. – Brush off solids and powders. ■ Remove all clothing to ensure that traces of the chemical do not remain trapped in shoes or folds of clothing where they can continue to burn. ■ Diluting and removing the chemicals should continue during transport, with extra attention given to guarding both the EMT and the patient from splashing and runoff.
R-63	Electrical Burns ■ Cause of death ■ Other damage	Special complications: electrical burns ■ Death caused through either ventricular fibrillation or asphyxia ■ The extent of the damage done may not be readily apparent at the time of injury but presents later as dysfunction of vital organs occurs. ■ If the myocardium is affected, potentially life-threatening cardiac dysrhythmias may occur.

- Because the true extent of the damage is impossible to evaluate at the scene, these patients need rapid transportation to the hospital. The EMTs should be prepared to provide CPR en route.

R-64

Burn Trauma Summary
- Primary considerations
- Management of thermal burns

Thermal burn management summary:
- Safety, scene, and situation
- Stop the burning process.
- Aggressively manage the patient's airway, breathing, burn wound care, and circulation.
- Treat any serious associated injuries.
- For patients in shock, early rapid transport to an appropriate facility takes precedence over actual care of the burn itself.
- If the patient is stable, the following steps can be taken to care for the burn:
  - Remove or cut away the patient's clothing, leaving only those pieces which adhere to the burn areas.
  - Remove all jewelry to eliminate heated metal from contacting the skin and to reduce problems which may be caused by edema.
  - Cover the burns with DRY clean sterile sheets. Wet dressings may be used with caution over no more than 10% of the patient's entire body surface area for pain relief on second degree burns. Monitor for hypothermia.
  - With second degree burns, the EMT should be careful to maintain the integrity of any blisters that have formed.

Patient assessment

- The trauma patient presents the EMT with a unique and complex challenge.
- The EMT must perform a solid, rapid assessment to find or rule out all life-threatening and serious conditions.
- The EMT must then correctly classify the patient as having either simple, isolated injuries or multisystem trauma.

Evaluate patient's condition

Patients with simple trauma need a complete assessment to uncover and identify all problems and to determine appropriate care for their injuries. The EMT has time to fully assess and monitor the patient and to provide safe, careful transportation to an appropriate medical facility.

Evaluate patient's condition

With multisystem trauma patients, the EMT must identify and focus on their critical needs:

- Aggressive airway management
- Ventilation with high FiO_2 to combat hypoxia
- Aggressive shock therapy to maintain adequate perfusion
- Key treatment steps include:
  - Preserving body temperature
  - Pneumatic antishock garment
  - Long backboard to provide rapid whole-body immobilization

Slide No.	Description	Lecture Content
		– Initiating at least two large-bore IV lines – Rapid packaging – Early transport to an appropriate trauma facility ■ Essential injury management depending on the patient's wounds include: – Chest decompression – Sealing of sucking chest or abdominal wounds – Controlling hemorrhage – Stabilization of flail segments
R-65	Key Considerations ■ Recognize critical needs of the patient ■ Efficiency of care ■ Aggressive intervention ■ Rapid packaging ■ Rapid transport ■ Continue treatment ■ Nearest appropriate hospital	Time is of the essence in the management of the multisystem trauma patient. ■ Within the "Platinum 10 Minutes" the EMT must: – Correctly identify the critical nature of the patient's injuries – Aggressively treat only those conditions which are immediately life threatening – Quickly package the patient – Rapidly initiate transportation to the nearest appropriate facility ■ Once en route, the patient can be evaluated with a cardiac monitor, and a more thorough secondary assessment can be conducted if time and the patient's condition allow. ■ It is the EMT's management of the first few minutes of prehospital care that often makes the difference between life and death for the critical trauma patient.
R-66	Title Slide	Trauma megatrends
R-67	Trauma Today and Tomorrow	This section will be changed as new research is done and new ideas in patient care are accepted or envisioned. This section will identify those current changes as well as the important things to look for in the future. The objective of this section is to provide an update at the basic or advanced levels about what is happening in the care of the trauma patient and what new things to look for.

R-68	PHTLS Trauma Update Objectives
	■ Current ATLS guidelines
	■ Controversial topics (PASG, IV, etc.)
	■ Possible changes based on available research
		There are three aspects to this section: One is to identify the new changes coming into the ATLS course that affect prehospital providers.
		  PHTLS has always been, and will be for the future, based upon the ATLS teachings. The guidelines in PHTLS will change with changes in ATLS through the close working relationship between the National Association of EMTs, its PHTLS Committee, and the American College of Surgeons Committee on Trauma.
		  The second and third aspects of this section will include items where new study is occurring as well as controversial topics.

Slide No.	Description	Lecture Content
R-69	Trends Multisystem Trauma Patient	Trends • Trauma prevention 　– Traumatic injury continues to exact a tremendous yearly toll on Americans. Both in terms of lives lost and disabilities sustained, the impact is economically and personally devastating. It is an often cited statistic that trauma accounts for more deaths in the 1 to 44-year-old age group than all other causes combined. The national response to this statistic has included the establishment of sophisticated trauma centers, the institution of systems for rapid transport of the trauma victim, and the support and production of voluminous research regarding optimal care for traumatic injuries.
R-70	Injury Prevention	– However, one area that has been largely ignored is the prevention of traumatic injury. Consequently, the Centers for Disease Control (CDC), through in-depth study and the foundation of various subcommittees, has set a "National Agenda for Injury Control in the 1990s." Through its position papers, the CDC has established injury prevention as a national priority and urges commitment to the same at the state and local level. As providers of prehospital and in-hospital care, it behooves all of us to educate our communities about trauma and trauma prevention. Specific topics highlighted include the following:
R-71	Motor Vehicle Injury Prevention • Requires stricter 　– Safety belt use 　– Helmet use 　– Child safety seat use 　– Enforcement of impaired driving laws 　– Guidelines for improved vehicle safety devices and designs • Improved vehicle safety devices and designs • Opposition to increased speed limits • Reduce availability and consumption of drugs and alcohol.	• Motor vehicle injury prevention 　– Stricter safety belt, helmet, and child safety seat laws 　– Stricter enforcement of impaired driving laws 　– Improved vehicle safety devices and designs 　– Opposition to increased speed limits and more stringent enforcement of existing limits 　– Support of a national agenda to reduce the promotion, availability, and consumption of drugs and alcohol
R-72	Prevention of Violence and Violent Injuries • Develop violence prevention and intervention programs (Safe Kids, etc.)	• Prevention of violence and violent injuries 　– Develop violence prevention and intervention programs, especially at the community level. 　– Improve the recognition, referral, treatment, and tracking of violent people and victims of violence.

Slide No.	Description	Lecture Content
	■ Improve recognition, referral, treatment, and tracking of victims of violence. ■ Increase awareness of and education about firearm safety	– Increase awareness of firearm safety. – Increase education regarding firearm safety.
R-73	Prevention of Violence and Violent Injuries ■ Reduce the use of drugs and alcohol by violent and potentially violent persons ■ Provide early childhood intervention programs. ■ Educate and protect potential victims of violent injury.	■ Reduce the use of drugs and alcohol by violent and potentially violent persons. ■ Provide early childhood intervention to educate and protect the potential victims and perpetrators of violent injury.
R-74	Home and Leisure Injury Prevention ■ Educate public about potential hazards in the home. ■ Enforce design standards to make home equipment safer. ■ Support community efforts in first aid and basic life support (BLS).	■ Home and leisure injury prevention (i.e., falls, burns, firearm injuries, drownings, etc.) – Educate the public about potential hazards in the home. – Enforce design standards to make home equipment safer. – Support community efforts to train citizens in first aid and basic life support.
R-75	Occupational Injury Prevention ■ Maintain federal standards of safety. ■ Reward injury prevention programs. ■ Establish injury surveillance systems. ■ Expand coverage of workers under federal programs.	■ Occupational injury prevention – Maintain federal standards of safety. – Reward injury prevention. – Establish injury surveillance systems. – Expand coverage of workers under federal programs.
R-76	Injury Prevention Should be Everyone's Goal.	The prevention of traumatic injury should be everyone's goal. As prehospital providers, we are often the first to arrive at the scene of an accident. Unfortunately by then, the injury has already occurred and our efforts are directed toward preventing further harm.

Slide No.	Description	Lecture Content

We all should think about involving our communities in a campaign to prevent traumatic injury. We should apply our experience and expertise to the development of programs that educate the public about ways to reduce the toll of traumatic injury and death.

R-77

Intraosseous Infusion

- Has become widely accepted standard for pediatric care
- Quick
- Relatively safe and easy to perform

Intraosseous infusion

- It is well known among prehospital providers that vascular access in children is often difficult, if not impossible. Lack of experience, a frenzied environment, heightened anxiety, and miniaturized anatomy all contribute to failure at IV access. The provider becomes frustrated and patient care can be compromised. For the past several years, intraosseous infusion has become widely accepted as an alternative to traditional peripheral IV access. Most prehospital providers are familiar with the procedure but many have not had the opportunity to use it. Consequently, this limited experience may make some providers reluctant to rapidly employ this option and instead to opt for repeated attempts at upper extremity sites.

  We all must realize that when done properly, intraosseous infusion is a quick, easy, and safe procedure. One must not delay gaining quick vascular access in the critically ill or injured child. If lack of experience and confidence is limiting use of this technique, then we must encourage more skills reviews and classes to teach it. Intraosseous infusion is a good, powerful tool in the prehospital setting.

R-78

Pulse Oximetry

Measures:

- Estimation of pulmonary oxygenation
- RBC oxygen saturation

Does not measure:

- Tissue oxygenation
- Oxygen delivery
- Aerobic versus anaerobic metabolism

- Pulse oximetry
  - The use of pulse oximetry has improved the capabilities of measuring tissue oxygen. However, pulse oximetry measures the oxygen saturation of the red cells, or the percentage of oxygen present in the available RBCs; it is not related to the PaO_2. The PaO_2 may be increased by dissolved oxygen in the bloodstream and decreased by a reduction in the number and volume of red blood cells without changing oxygen saturation or each individual cell.
- Using an analogy, pulse oximetry measures how full the trucks carrying the oxygen are but does not measure the amount of oxygen that is actually delivered to the tissues. To continue the example, if through hemorrhage a large quantity of RBCs have been lost, only a very few trucks are available. They all can be 100% full but not deliver an adequate amount of oxygen. Think of pulse oximetry as the adequacy of the lung function but not the delivery system.

R-79

Ventilation Evaluation
Hospital care: $PaCO_2$
Prehospital: respiratory rate

- 12–20 per minute = good

- As the ventilatory rate drops, the capabilities of the lungs to provide adequate elimination of carbon dioxide by way of ventilation also decreases. One can estimate the acid load in the form of CO_2 by counting the respiratory rate. (12 to 20 = good; above 20 = questionable; above 30 = bad).

Slide No.	Description	Lecture Content
	■ >20 = questionable ■ <10 = bad	**Conclusion:** When properly interpreted, pulse oximetry represents a significant advance in identifying hypoxia and in monitoring the effectiveness of ventilation and oxygenation in the field.

R-80	Blood-borne Infections
	■ Hepatitis is still more hazardous to EMS than the HIV/AIDS virus
	  – Less contamination required
	  – One contact may infect
	  – Hepatitis B vaccines are available
	  – Death rate among health care personnel annually is much higher than for HIV/AIDS
		• Blood-borne infections
		  – Each year 250 or more healthcare workers die of hepatitis.

R-81	Blood-borne Infections—Prevention
	■ Prior immunization
	■ Body surface isolation (BSI) skin protection
	■ Wash carefully after contact
	■ Consult physician after significant contact
		• It is much easier to get hepatitis than AIDS. Therefore, one must work to prevent contact. Once such contact has been made, immediate treatment is necessary. The best approach is to obtain an active immunization with the vaccination prior to contact.
		  – Ensure prior immunization
		  – Protect skin from contact with body fluids.
		  – Wash skin with peroxide, alcohol, or strong soap after contact.
		  – Percutaneous contamination should be immediately checked by the emergency department and appropriate local protocols followed for treatment.

R-82	Patient Movement ■ Logroll only when necessary ■ Roll only as high as required ■ Use scoop when possible	• Spine fractures – Recent literature suggests that logrolling a patient to 90° to place a backboard may produce unwanted movement to the spine. A preferable approach would be to lift the patient onto a longboard with a scoop stretcher. More study is needed of different logroll methods, straddle slide, and scoop to resolve this issue. Until these are available, it would be prudent to logroll only when necessary and use the scoop when possible.
R-83	Controversies	• Topics covered have been identified as controversial but may still be beneficial when caring for certain patients.

R-84	Pneumatic Antishock Garment (PASG)
	■ Increase systemic vascular resistance
	■ Performs autotransfusion
	■ Tamponades bleeding
	■ Stabilizes fractures
		• Pneumatic Antishock Garment (PASG)
		• For more than a decade, the PASG has been standard prehospital equipment. The theory supporting its use in traumatic hypotension is based on the following four physiologic mechanisms:
		  – Increase systemic vascular resistance
		  – Cause autotransfusion of blood from the lower extremities
		  – Tamponade bleeding vessels
		  – Stabilize fractures

Slide No.	Description	Lecture Content

R-85

PASG limitations:
- Prolong scene time
- Cause metabolic acidosis and/or compartment syndrome
- Limit physical examination
- Worsen thoracic injury outcomes

However, in recent years the usefulness of the PASG has been questioned. Some researchers maintain that application of the PASG can prolong scene time, thereby delaying arrival at a trauma center and subsequent definitive operative intervention. Other authors have suggested that the PASG can cause metabolic acidosis and/or compartment syndrome if left on for a long time. Furthermore, the PASG can prevent adequate examination of abdominal and lower extremity injuries as a route of fluid resuscitation. Perhaps most troubling is the recent literature, which charges that use of the PASG in thoracic injury actually worsens outcome.

Current prehospital standards of care continue to support the use of the PASG in the patient with traumatic hypotension. However, in light of recent research and the feeling of some trauma and emergency physicians, the future trend may well be away from routine application of the PASG. Rapid transport and definitive care remain the cornerstones of successful trauma management.

R-86

Hypertonic Saline
- Replenishes intravascular space and circulating volume
- Causes rapid fluid shift from intracellular and interstitial compartments into intravascular space
- Current evidence: Does not support routine use of hypertonic solutions

- Hypertonic saline
- The human body is approximately 60% water. Two-thirds of the fluid is in the intracellular space and one-third is extracellular. The extracellular compartment is further divided into the interstitial and intravascular spaces. The immediate goal of posttraumatic fluid resuscitation is replenishment of the intravascular space and therefore of circulating volume.

Routine prehospital and in-hospital trauma resuscitation fluids are normal saline solutions and Ringer's lactate. These are isotonic fluids which rapidly equilibrate with the total extracellular space. Consequently, intravascular volume is replaced.

It has been theorized that a solution of hypertonic saline with or without dextran would, via osmotic forces, cause a rapid fluid shift from the intracellular and interstitial compartments into the intravascular space. Recruitment of this fluid into the intravascular space could cause an immediate, if transient, increase in available circulating volume. Posttraumatic shock could be averted or at least delayed. Several studies have been undertaken to assess the effect of prehospital and in-hospital administration of small-volume hypertonic saline and saline/dextran in initial posttraumatic resuscitation. The weight of the current evidence does not support the routine use of hypertonic solutions in trauma resuscitation because statistical improvement in patient outcome has not been conclusively demonstrated. Some authors note improvement and some did note a trend (without statistical significance) toward decreased mortality/morbidity in the trauma victims treated with hypertonic fluids. However, other studies support that hypertonic solutions can actually increase bleeding (via vasodilation) in a nontamponaded vessel, leading to worsening and hemorrhagic shock.

Slide No.	Description	Lecture Content
R-87	Hypertonic Saline • May prove useful: posttraumatic hypotension and head injury • Hypertonic solutions may have some potential benefit	One area in which hypertonic solutions may prove useful is in the initial resuscitation of the multiple-injured patient with concurrent posttraumatic hypotension and head injury. The theory maintains that limiting the volume of resuscitation fluids required to restore hemodynamic stability will diminish the increase in the intracranial pressure typically seen in the head-injured patient. This could improve long-term outcome in the patient who survives his or her initial injuries. To summarize, hypertonic solutions as initial small-volume resuscitation fluids have demonstrated some potential positive benefit. However, studies have not been conclusive enough to warrant a change in current prehospital and in-hospital practices.
R-88	Intubation/Airway Management	• Intubation/airway management
R-89	Double-lumen Airway Devices	Pharyngeal-tracheal lumen (PTL) • Airway management remains an absolute priority in the treatment of the trauma victim. Standard airway adjuncts are the oropharyngeal and nasopharyngeal airways and the endotracheal tube. The esophageal obturator airway has been widely criticized and is no longer considered a reliable tool in airway management. A new airway, the pharyngeal tracheal lumen (PTL), has recently been introduced in this country. It consists of two tubes; one long and one short. The long tube is blindly inserted into the mouth and past the pharynx. It lodges in either the trachea or the esophagus. Blowing up a balloon on the distal end of the tube, listening for breath sounds, and watching for chest wall rise helps determine whether the balloon has occluded the esophagus or trachea. The patient is then ventilated via various proximal ports, depending on the site of the long tube. A second balloon is blown up in the patient's mouth, which occludes the oropharynx. This aids adequate distal ventilation by preventing retrograde leaks and helps secure the entire PTL in place.
R-90	Advantages of ETC/PTL • Ease of use • Placement done by blind technique • Provides a more definitive airway than basic techniques • May be placed in the esophagus or trachea • High success and low complication rates • Can be placed without C-spine manipulation	Advantages of the PTL include blind placement with the head in a neutral position, thus permitting its use in trauma patients. It does not require a mask, so adequate face-mask seal is not a problem. Presumably it can be performed with less training than is required for endotracheal intubation.

Slide No.	Description	Lecture Content

R-91	Disadvantages of ETC/PTL
	
	• Limited studies in pre-hospital use
	• Cannot be used in children or adults under 4 feet in height
	• Not nearly as definitive as ET intubation
	• Contraindications
	  – Presence of a gag reflex
	  – Conscious or unconscious and breathing patients
	  – Obstructed airway
	  – Caustic indigestion or esophageal disease
	• Definitive studies are still required to validate its efficacy
		However, several disadvantages exist as well. The PTL tube looks complicated and is cumbersome with multiple tubes and ports. Placement is relatively simple but confirmation can be difficult and fraught with complication. Breath sounds can be difficult or impossible to hear, the chest wall rise may not be obvious, and the wrong ports can inadvertently be used.

R-92	Endotracheal Intubation Remains the Airway of Choice	In conclusion, while the PTL has several attractive features, it is not without risks. Consequently it has not been embraced with unequivocal enthusiasm by the prehospital community. Few services use it at all, and most do not have plans to adopt it in the near future. Endotracheal intubation remains the airway of choice in the prehospital and in-hospital environment.

R-93	Summary
	
	• Trauma prevention
	
	• Intraosseous infusion
	
	• Pulse oximetry
	
	• Blood-borne infections
		Summary
		After covering such a diverse group of topics, a summary and some conclusions are useful.
		
		• Trauma prevention
		  – Has been largely ignored
		  – Should be everyone's goal
		  – Apply our experience and expertise to help educate public
		• Intraosseous infusion
		  – Becoming more widely accepted
		  – Offers a quick access in pediatric patients
		• Pulse oximetry
		  – Measures estimation of pulmonary oxygenation
		  – Measures RBC oxygen saturation
		  – Use when available
		• Blood-borne infections
		  – Hepatitis more common than AIDS
		  – Get immunization
		  – Use body surface isolation (BSI)
		  – Report possible contamination immediately

Slide No.	Description	Lecture Content
	▪ Spine fractures	▪ Spine fractures and patient movement – Logrolling may produce unwanted movement of spine – Use scoop stretcher when possible
	▪ Pneumatic antishock garment	▪ Pneumatic antishock garment – Continued support of use in prehospital setting – Rapid transport and definitive care remain crucial
	▪ Hypertonic saline	▪ Hypertonic saline – Some potential benefit – No change currently
	▪ Double-lumen airway devices	▪ Double-lumen airway devices – Advantages – Disadvantages – Endotracheal intubation remains airway of choice

SECTION V

Administration

Course Planning Schedule: A Guide for the Course Coordinator

COURSE COORDINATOR SCHEDULE ACTIVITY FORM

Course #: _____   Dates: _____

TIME FRAME	STATUS (Y OR N)	ACTIVITY
90 days	_____	Identify date, site, faculty, and medical director.
	_____	Identify maximum number of students and marketing strategy.
	_____	Forward Course Planning Form to the regional or state coordinator with proposed budget and faculty list.
	_____	Secure lecture room and skill station breakout rooms (confirm in writing).
	_____	Reserve hotel accommodations (if required).
	_____	Apply for CME credit.
	_____	Reserve audiovisual equipment.
	_____	Draft brochure and mailing list.
	_____	Identify skill station equipment.
When course approval is granted	_____	Receive written verification from state coordinator and/or national office.
	_____	Print and distribute brochures.
	_____	Confirm faculty.
	_____	Receive course materials from PHTLS International Office.
	_____	Process and notify students.
	_____	Provide faculty with schedule, location, and educational outlines.
	_____	Communicate with affiliate faculty if applicable.
	_____	Confirm moulage technician.
	_____	Arrange for meals and breaks.

TIME FRAME	STATUS (Y OR N)	ACTIVITY
30 days	_____	Arrange for patient models.
	_____	Prepare directional signs.
	_____	Order disposable supplies.
	_____	Reconfirm equipment arrangements.
	_____	Mail final materials to students.
	_____	Mail slides and outlines to the faculty.
1 week before course	_____	Reconfirm lecture and skill station rooms.
	_____	Reconfirm faculty and patient models.
	_____	Prepare student rotation groups.
	_____	Confirm final arrangements with the affiliate faculty if applicable.
	_____	Assemble course written materials.
2 days before course	_____	Collect all equipment and supplies.
	_____	Prepare name tags for faculty and students.
	_____	Remind faculty of assignments.
	_____	Reconfirm refreshments and lunch.
	_____	Prepare CME certificates (if required).
1 day before course	_____	Ensure that rooms are set up.
	_____	Check all equipment.
	_____	Meet with course faculty and PHTLS affiliate faculty if applicable.

TIME FRAME	STATUS (Y OR N)	ACTIVITY
Days of course	_____	Ensure that refreshments are available.
	_____	Place directional signs throughout the facility.
	_____	Check rooms.
	_____	Collect slides from lecture faculty.
	_____	Collect evaluations.
	_____	Complete course roster and summary.
After the course	_____	Clean and return equipment.
	_____	Return slides to the PHTLS International Office (if on loan).
	_____	Write thank you letters.
	_____	Submit postcourse paperwork and surcharge check to the PHTLS International Office.

Precourse Forms

NAEMT PREHOSPITAL TRAUMA LIFE SUPPORT COURSE
COURSE PLANNING AND APPROVAL FORM*

Send to: PHTLS International Office
408 Monroe Street
Clinton, MS 39056

I. SPONSOR IDENTIFICATION   REGION: _____

   A. Local Sponsoring Organization   _____
      Mailing Address   _____
      City/State (Prov.)/Zip Code   _____
      Telephone Number   _____

   B. Proposed Course Coordinator   _____
      Title   _____
      Phone (Office)   _____
      Mailing Address   _____
      City/State (Prov.)/Zip Code   _____

   C. Proposed Course Medical Director   _____
      Background   _____
      ATLS Instructor?   _____ Yes _____ No
      Mailing Address   _____
      City/State (Prov.)/Zip Code   _____

II. NATIONAL COURSE # _____   STATE COURSE # _____

   A. Facility Name   _____
      Address   _____
      City/State (Prov.)/Zip Code   _____
      Contact Person   _____
      Phone   _____
      Exact class location within facility   _____

   B. Proposed Course Dates: Start Date: _____ End Date: _____

   C. Expected # of students:
      _____ Basic Provider   _____ Advance Provider
      _____ Basic Provider Instr.   _____ Advance Provider Instr.
      _____ Basic I/C   _____ Advance I/C
      _____ Basic Refresher   _____ Advance Refresher
      _____ Instructor Update   _____ Military

   D. Attach proposed course budget (be as complete and specific as possible).

   E. Attach proposed course faculty list, including medical background and lecture/skill station assignments.

   F. Slides needed?   _____ Yes _____ No

*Must be received by regional/state coordinator 90 days in advance of proposed course dates.

G. We agree that the NAEMT regional faculty member on-site is the final authority on the conduct of the course and must be consulted in writing for approval before any alterations in schedule, etc. may be made.

_____   _____
Date   Responsible Officer of Host Organization

_____   _____
Date   Proposed Course Coordinator

_____   _____
Date   Proposed Course Medical Director

DO NOT WRITE BELOW THIS LINE

Received _____   Approved _____

State COT chairperson_____

Sponsor OK: REG COORD _____   COT _____   Date _____

CMD OK   _____   _____   _____

Site OK   _____   _____   _____

Date OK   _____   _____   _____

Affiliate faculty assigned, as necessary _____

PREHOSPITAL TRAUMA LIFE SUPPORT
COURSE BUDGET

Course date(s): _____   Sponsor: _____

Submitted by: _____   Date: _____

EXPENSES

Personnel
Lecturers _____
Skill station instructors _____
Victims/moulage _____
Secretarial support _____
Other _____

Affiliate Faculty (as applicable)
Travel _____
Lodging _____
Meals _____

Facilities
Facility charge _____
Meals (lunch, etc.) _____
Refreshments _____
Other _____

Materials, Equipment, and Supplies
Equipment rental _____
Expendable supplies _____
Printing/duplication _____
Brochures _____
Postage _____
Other _____
Textbooks _____

PHTLS Surcharge
Provider: $15 × _____ _____
Instructor: $15 × _____ _____
Refresher: $10 × _____ _____
Miscellaneous _____

TOTAL EXPENSES _____

REVENUES
Tuition fee $ _____ × _____ students _____
Textbooks sold _____
Meal(s) fee (if charged) _____
Other _____

TOTAL REVENUES _____
NET _____

Forms for Use During the Course

PREHOSPITAL TRAUMA LIFE SUPPORT ANSWER SHEET

Pre _____ Post _____   Name: _____

National Course #: _____ State Course #: _____

Course Location: _____

Dates of Course: _____

Social Security #: _____ Test #: _____

ANSWER SHEET

1. A B C D	26. A B C D
2. A B C D	27. A B C D
3. A B C D	28. A B C D
4. A B C D	29. A B C D
5. A B C D	30. A B C D
6. A B C D	31. A B C D
7. A B C D	32. A B C D
8. A B C D	33. A B C D
9. A B C D	34. A B C D
10. A B C D	35. A B C D
11. A B C D	36. A B C D
12. A B C D	37. A B C D
13. A B C D	38. A B C D
14. A B C D	39. A B C D
15. A B C D	40. A B C D
16. A B C D	41. A B C D
17. A B C D	42. A B C D
18. A B C D	43. A B C D
19. A B C D	44. A B C D
20. A B C D	45. A B C D
21. A B C D	46. A B C D
22. A B C D	47. A B C D
23. A B C D	48. A B C D
24. A B C D	49. A B C D
25. A B C D	50. A B C D

PREHOSPITAL TRAUMA LIFE SUPPORT
STUDENT REGISTRATION FORM

Note: Please Print

National Course #: _____   State Course #: _____

Date: _____   Social Security #: _____

Name:_____

Street: _____

City: _____   State: _____   Zip: _____

Home Phone #: (___) _____   Work Phone #: (___) _____

EMT-BASIC _____   EMT-INT _____   EMT-P _____   RN _____   MD _____

Other (Specify):_____

Expiration Date of Certificate or License: _____

State Issued: _____

National Registry _____   NREMT-BASIC _____   NREMT-INT _____   NREMT-P _____

Previous Courses Successfully Completed:

PHTLS BASIC _____   PHTLS I/C _____   PHTLS REFRESHER _____

BTLS _____   BTLS I/C _____

Location of Last Course Taken:_____

Date of Last Course: _____   NAEMT Member: Yes _____   No _____

Student Signature:_____

FACULTY/STAFF ONLY TO WRITE IN THIS AREA:

Current State Certificate, Documented _____ (Staff Initials)

Previous Provider/Refresher Course, Documented _____ (Staff Initials)

Pretest Score _____   Posttest Score _____

Final Assessment _____

REFRESHER COURSE SKILL STATION SUMMARY SHEET

Student Name: _____

COURSE FACULTY ONLY TO WRITE BELOW THIS LINE

SKILL STATIONS (Faculty to initial appropriate spaces)

	If Assessment Leader	Passed	Needs Retest	Passed Retest	Failed Retest
#1 Patient Assessment "A"	____	____	____	____	____
#2 Patient Assessment "B"	____	____	____	____	____
#3 Airway and Ventilation	____	____	____	____	____
#4 Advanced Airway (Only Advanced Personnel)	____	____	____	____	____
#5 Spine "A" Logrolls and Standing Longboard	____	____	____	____	____
#6 Spine "B" Rapid Extrication	____	____	____	____	____

Course coordinator to fill in items below:

Needs Remediation/Retest of Stations: _____

Written Test Score: _____   Needs Retest of Written: _____

Passed All Stations (Initially or Retest): _____

Passed Written Test (Initially or Retest): _____

Passed Refresher: _____   New Certificate Issued, Expiration Date: _____

Failed to Meet Requirements: _____   Letter Sent: _____

_____
Refresher Course Coordinator Signature

PHTLS BASELINE SKILL EVALUATION SHEET

Date: _____   Group: _____

Evaluator and Patient: _____

Start Time: _____   End Time: _____

Elapsed Time:

Y	N	Late	____:____	Scene Safety
Y	N	Late	____:____	LOC
Y	N	Late	____:____	Manual C-spine
Y	N	Late	____:____	Airway
Y	N	Late	____:____	Breathing
Y	N	Late	____:____	Pulse
Y	N	Late	____:____	Bleeding
Y	N	Late	____:____	Exposure
Y	N	Late	____:____	Breath Sounds
Y	N	Late	____:____	Skin Quality
Y	N	Late	____:____	Capillary Refill
Y	N	Late	____:____	Rapid Extrication
Y	N	Late	____:____	Secure to Board
Y	N	Late	____:____	High-Flow Oxygen
Y	N	Late	____:____	Vital Signs
Y	N	Late	____:____	Transportation
Y	N	Late	____:____	Tier with ALS/Air
Y	N	Late	____:____	PASG
Y	N	Late	____:____	C-collar Application
Y	N	Late	____:____	Focused Exam
Y	N	Late	____:____	Detailed Exam
Y	N	Late	____:____	Noncritical Tx
Y	N	Patient Survives		

First Vital Signs:

Pulse: _____

B/P: _____

Resp: _____

Skin: _____

Time: _____

Second Vital Signs:

Pulse: _____

B/P: _____

Resp: _____

Skin: _____

Time: _____

Third Vital Signs:

Pulse: _____

B/P: _____

Resp: _____

Skin: _____

Time: _____

NOTES:

BASELINE DETERMINATIONS
EVALUATION FLOW SHEET

Group: _____ Total time at scene: _____

1 to 3
minutes:

3 to 6
minutes:

6 to 10
minutes:

Evalutor(s): _____

NOTE: This form is to document the student's general activity during the scenario.

SHEET TO BE USED FOR ALL FINAL ASSESSMENT STATIONS

FINAL ASSESSMENT STATION #: _____

EVALUATION FLOW SHEET

Group: _____ Total time at scene: _____

1 to 3
minutes:

3 to 6
minutes:

6 to 10
minutes:

Evaluator(s): _____

_____

NOTE: This form is to document the student's general activity during the scenario.

PREHOSPITAL TRAUMA LIFE SUPPORT
COURSE SUMMARY EVALUATION

National Course #: _____   Course Location: _____

COURSE SUMMARY EVALUATION*

1. How well organized was the entire program?	1 2 3
2. To what extent did the program meet your needs?	1 2 3
3. Did the program meet the course objectives?	1 2 3
4. What is your overall evaluation of the program?	1 2 3
5. In general, how appropriate were the program handouts?	1 2 3
6. In general, how appropriate were the audiovisuals?	1 2 3
7. In general, was the level of material presented appropriate to your level of care?	1 2 3
8. To what extent will the information presented be of value to you?	1 2 3
9. Do you feel that your application of practical skills has improved as a result of this course?	1 2 3
10. If present, how well did the affiliate faculty represent PHTLS and the NAEMT?	1 2 3
11. How well were you informed about NAEMT and the benefits of membership?	1 2 3

12. What was the best or most helpful part of the program for you?

_____

_____

13. What was the worst or least helpful part of the program for you?

_____

_____

14. How beneficial were the skill stations?

Baselines	1 2 3	Rapid Extrication	1 2 3
Airway	1 2 3	Spinal Stabilization	1 2 3
Pediatric Assessment and Immobilization	1 2 3	Assessment	1 2 3
Final Assessment	1 2 3		

15. Would you recommend this course to others?   Yes _____ No _____

16. General comments:

_____

_____

1–ABOVE AVERAGE
2–AVERAGE
3–BELOW AVERAGE

*Must be given to regional or state coordinator

PREHOSPITAL TRAUMA LIFE SUPPORT
LECTURER EVALUATION FORM*

Name (Optional): _____

Topic: _____

Presenter: _____

How Would You Rate This Presentation?

1. Organization of presentation   1 2 3
2. Knowledge of content   1 2 3
3. Outline handout   1 2 3
4. Audiovisual materials   1 2 3
5. Material presented   1 2 3
6. Blend of theory and practice   1 2 3
7. Presentation length   1 2 3
8. My knowledge was increased.   1 2 3
9. What part of the presentation was **most** helpful or informative to you?

_____

_____

_____

10. What part of the presentation was **least** helpful or informative to you?

_____

_____

_____

11. General comments:

_____

_____

_____

1–ABOVE AVERAGE
2–AVERAGE
3–BELOW AVERAGE

*This form is optional and can be given to lecture faculty.

PREHOSPITAL TRAUMA LIFE SUPPORT
REFRESHER COURSE EVALUATION FORM

Course Location: _____   Date: _____

Certification: _____   Course #: _____

1—ABOVE AVERAGE   2—AVERAGE   3—BELOW AVERAGE

1. What is your overall evaluation of the course?	1	2	3
2. How well did "Managing the Multisystem Trauma Patient" review the material?	1	2	3
3. How valuable was "Pediatric Trauma"?	1	2	3
4. How valuable was "Trauma of the Elderly"?	1	2	3
5. How well did "Megatrends" present "What's New, What's Changed, What's Controversial"?	1	2	3
6. Overall, how would you rate the lecture faculty?	1	2	3

7. How well did each station review and measure your ability in the required skills?

Skill Station #1—Assessment "A"	1	2	3
Skill Station #2—Assessment "B"	1	2	3
Skill Station #3—Airway and Ventilation	1	2	3
Skill Station #4—Advanced Airway	1	2	3
Skill Station #5—Spine Skills	1	2	3
Skill Station #6—Rapid Extrication	1	2	3
8. Overall, how would you rate skill station instuctors?	1	2	3
9. How would you rate the PHTLS refresher course design, sequence, and content?	1	2	3
10. How would you rate the organization of the course you just finished?	1	2	3
11. How would you rate the facilities?	1	2	3

12. What was the **BEST** PART of the course? _____

_____

13. What was the **WORST** PART of the course? _____

_____

14. Other comments: _____

_____

FINAL EVALUATION STATION SCENARIO FLOW SHEET

Group Number: _____   Group Leader: _____

Evaluator: _____   Scenario Number: _____

Beginning Time: _____   Ending Time: _____

Completed		
Yes	**No**	**Assessment and Treatment**
		Identify safe scene
		Proper body substance protection
		Perform complete initial (primary) assessment
		Level of consciousness/response
		Airway
		Breathing
		Ventilation/air exchange
		Circulation/perfusion
		Pulse
		External hemorrhage control
		Skin conditions
		Exposure of all critical body areas for assessment
		Properly identify critical or noncritical trauma patient
		Use of appropriate spinal immobilization technique(s)
		Proper use of padding/buttress material
		Identification of all life-threatening injuries
		Proper treatment of life-threatening injuries
		Performed only lifesaving treatment(s) while on-scene
		Timely transport when indicated
		Appropriate level trauma facility when indicated
		Identification of all noncritical injuries
		Proper treatment performed en route
		Complete detailed (secondary) assessment when indicated
		Completed scenario within 10 minutes on-scene time
		Reassessment of patient's condition
		Safety observed throughout scenario
		Worked together as a team

Successful Station Completion: Yes _____   No _____

Any mark(s) within the critical criteria area would indicate the need for the group to repeat the station. Only mark those comments that apply to the scenario. Please document rationale for any checked critical criteria in the notation area.

Critical Criteria

_____ Failure to utilize proper body substance isolation techniques

_____ Failure to identify safe scene

_____ Failure to perform adequate/complete initial (primary) assessment

_____ Failure to identify all life-threatening injuries/conditions

_____ Failure to immediately treat life-threatening injuries/conditions

_____ Failure to identify critical patient based on assessment

_____ Performed unnecessary treatment on-scene

_____ Performed detailed (secondary) assessment before initial assessment

_____ Failure to complete a detailed (secondary) assessment

_____ Failure to assess and treat noncritical injuries

_____ Failure to provide timely transport to an appropriate level trauma facility

_____ Failure to reassess the patient's condition

_____ Failure to perform scenario in a safe manner

_____ Failure to perform scenario in a team fashion

_____ Failure to complete scenario within 10 minutes of on-scene time

Notations:

_____

_____

_____

_____

Postcourse Forms

PREHOSPITAL TRAUMA LIFE SUPPORT
COURSE ROSTER

National Course #: _____   State Course #: _____   Course Date: _____

Location/sponsor: _____

City, State, Zip: _____

LEVEL OF COURSE: ADVANCED PROVIDER (AP)
                          ADVANCED INSTRUCTOR (AI)
                          ADVANCED REFRESHER (AR)
                          BASIC PROVIDER (BP)
                          BASIC INSTRUCTOR (BI)
                          BASIC REFRESHER (BR)

#	Student Name	Student Address	Social Security #	Phone Number	NAEMT Member (Y or N)	Course Level	Status Pass or Fail
1							
2							
3							
4							
5							
6							
7							
8							
9							
10							
11							
12							
13							
14							
15							

#	Student Name	Student Address	Social Security #	Phone Number	NAEMT Member (Y or N)	Course Level	Status Pass or Fail
16							
17							
18							
19							
20							
21							
22							
23							
24							
25							
26							
27							
28							
29							
30							
31							
32							
33							
34							
35							
36							

This PHTLS course was conducted as prescribed by the NAEMT/PHTLS Program.

_____ _____ _____
Course Coordinator   Course Medical Director   Affiliate Faculty
                                                           (if present)

PREHOSPITAL TRAUMA LIFE SUPPORT
INSTRUCTOR ROSTER

Course Date: _____   National Course Number: _____   State Course Number: _____

Course Sponsor/Location: _____

Address: _____

Course Coordinator: _____   Course Medical Director: _____

Instructor Name (Check ☐ if being monitored)	S.S. #	Mailing Address	Phone #	PHTLS Certified Instructor
☐				Y N
☐				Y N
☐				Y N
☐				Y N
☐				Y N
☐				Y N
☐				Y N
☐				Y N
☐				Y N
☐				Y N
☐				Y N

References

Bova B: Abdominal trauma lecture, Oklahoma PHTLS instructor course, Oklahoma City, 1986.

Davies IK: *Instructional technique,* New York, 1981, McGraw-Hill.

Foley R, Smilansky J: *Teaching techniques: a handbook for health professionals,* New York, 1980, McGraw-Hill.

Gardner H: *Frames of mind: the theory of multiple intelligences,* New York, 1985, Basic Books.

Laird D: *Approaches to training and development,* ed 2, Reading, Mass, 1985, Addison-Wesley.

Margolis F, Bell C: *Instructing for results,* Minneapolis, 1986, University Associates, San Diego and Lakewood Publications.

McConnel B: Instructional techniques lecture, PHTLS instructor course, Denver, 1986.

Parvensky CA: *Teaching EMS: an educator's guide to improved EMS instruction,* St Louis, 1995, JEMS Communications, Mosby Lifeline.

Prehospital Trauma Life Support Committee of the National Association of EMTs: *PHTLS basic and advanced instructor manual,* ed 3, St Louis, 1995, Mosby.

Prehospital Trauma Life Support Committee of the National Association of EMTs: *PHTLS Instructor slides,* St Louis, 1995, Mosby.

Shimamoto R: Instruction techniques lecture, PHTLS instructor course, French Camp, Calif, 1990.

NOTES

NOTES

NOTES